DOUBLE YOGA

Ganga White is an outstanding teacher and exponent of Yoga. He is president of the White Lotus Foundation, founder of the highly successful Center for Yoga in Los Angeles, and the originator of the Double Yoga system. Since 1966 he has spent his full time studying, teaching, and speaking on Yoga. He has trained hundreds of Yoga teachers and lived in India, where he visited remote monasteries and learning centers. He studied with many world-renowned teachers, including Venkatesa, B. K. S. Iyengar, and J. Krishnamurti. Mr. White has founded Yoga centers in major cities of the United States and for five years served as the vice president of the International Sivananda Yoga Vedanta Society. He has received the teaching title of *Yoga Acharya* three times—from the Sivananda Ashram; the Yoga Vedanta Forest University, Rishikesh, Himalayas; and the Yoga Niketan in India. He is certified in Homeopathy and Naturopathy. Mr. White's achievements and contributions to the field of Yoga have earned him the rare, honored title of *Yogiraj,* King of Yogis. He lives in Santa Barbara, California.

Anna Forrest is vice president of the White Lotus Foundation and senior instructor at the Center for Yoga in Los Angeles, where she received her training with Ganga White. She has studied Yoga in the United States and India and with B. K. S. Iyengar. Ms. Forrest has demonstrated Yoga on television in the United States and Japan and is certified in Homeopathy.

Poses by
GANGA WHITE and ANNA FORREST

Photographs by Michael Chesser

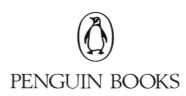

PENGUIN BOOKS

GANGA WHITE with ANNA FORREST

DoubleYoga

A New System for Total Body Health

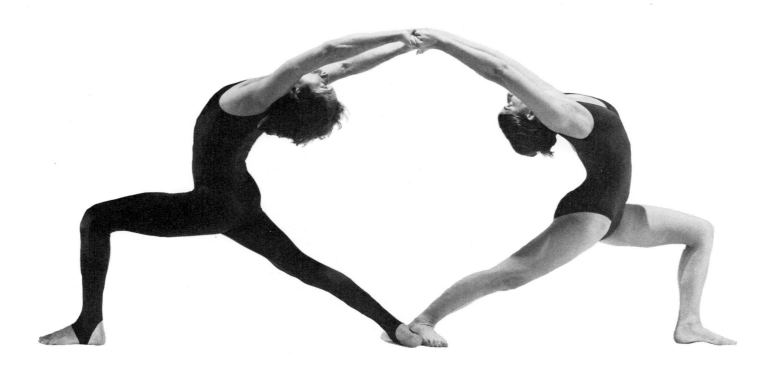

Penguin Books Ltd, Harmondsworth,
Middlesex, England
Penguin Books, 625 Madison Avenue,
New York, New York 10022, U.S.A.
Penguin Books Australia Ltd, Ringwood,
Victoria, Australia
Penguin Books Canada Limited, 2801 John Street,
Markham, Ontario, Canada L3R 1B4
Penguin Books (N.Z.) Ltd, 182–190 Wairau Road,
Auckland 10, New Zealand

First published 1981

LIBRARY OF CONGRESS CATALOGING IN PUBLICATION DATA
White, Ganga.
Double yoga.
(Penguin handbooks)
Includes index.
1. Yoga, Hatha. I. Title.
RA781.7.W49   613.7′046   81-7327
ISBN 0 14 046.505 7   AACR2

Printed in the United States of America by
Capital City Press, Inc., Montpelier, Vermont
Set in Fototronic Garamond

Designed by Ann Gold

To All Those Who Grow Beyond the
Limitations of Tradition

George White
3/21/8r

Contents

Acknowledgments

First I would like to express my appreciation to Yogini Anna Forrest. She has been of immeasurable assistance in developing the art and text of this book. Her hard work and dedication to Yoga are apparent in her degree of mastery. It is a joy and a privilege to work with her.

I also owe great appreciation to Michael Chesser, a talented and sensitive photographer with an eye for detail. His Yogic training gave him the necessary insight to take these technical photographs, and his good nature and cheerful manner made a difficult task a joyful and illuminating experience. Mike's artistry and sense of beauty are expressed in the photographs he created.

A special acknowledgment goes to Yogi B. K. S. Iyengar. Mr. Iyengar has made a valuable contribution to the science of Yoga. A number of the positions in this book have their roots in *asanas* developed by Mr. Iyengar.

Finally I would like to take this opportunity to express my deepest gratitude to the many Yogis and teachers I have studied with and to those who have handed and expanded this remarkable art down through the millennia. From teacher to student they gave a science that bestows great joy, freedom from suffering and ailments, and physical splendor. Salutations to those Yogis!

GANGA WHITE

Double Yoga

Welcome to Double Yoga

The word *Yoga* means union or reintegration, and the science of Yoga is grounded in the importance of achieving an integration of body, mind, and spirit so that one can live and act in harmony with all life.

In our complex world life has lost its simplicity. We face deep problems and immense challenges on every frontier, but oddly, though there is no shortage of "solutions," change doesn't come. Perhaps solutions and formulas are not the answer. Perhaps what is needed is a transformation of the human mind so that we can see clearly, maintain a quiet mind and sensitive body, and awaken to compassion, love, and intelligence. The teachings of Yoga encourage this transformation.

A vital, healthy body is the most basic prerequisite for one's journey in life. Hatha Yoga has come to be recognized as a superior form of physical culture for people of all ages, an enjoyable, noncompetitive way to total well-being. The word *Hatha* (pronounced *hah*-tah) comes from *ha,* meaning sun, and *tha,* meaning moon, and denotes the polarization of energy in the body. Hatha Yoga is the science of understanding the body in the fullest sense. It is unique in that it harmonizes physical, mental, and emotional functions. We now know that the patterns of modern life cause tension, anxiety, and premature physical degeneration. Yoga reestablishes the primal relationship between body and mind and restores the organism's balance. The body of a Hatha Yogi is supple, agile, alert, sensitive, and has abundant energy. In such a body the mind can reach and manifest its fullest potential.

Yoga originated thousands of years ago in India. Double Yoga is an exciting new development of the art. It is not meant to replace individual Yoga, but rather to add a new dimension to an ancient art. In practicing Yoga with another person, you are able to pull against your partner to get more stretch and effect in the poses. In some positions you will find it easier to maintain the correct balance, and in all the poses you will develop sensitivity and attunement to your partner. Although the photographs in the book show a man and a woman, the poses can be done just as easily by two men or two women. They can be adapted to varying sizes, abilities, and flexibilities of the partners. The body is a miraculous apparatus that can mold and adjust to give just the right support and force necessary to assist in accomplishing a movement or mastering a pose. There is an energy exchange when two people work together—it becomes easier to concentrate and hold the positions, attention is heightened, and you will be able to do things you could not possibly do alone. And there is great beauty in moving in rhythm and harmony with another person.

When two people hold a pose together, each partner experiences more energy than he or she contributes and many subtle lessons of relationship are demonstrated. Each learns how to give and take, to brace and embrace, and to literally bend over backward to assist the other. The partners learn to communicate nonverbally, to flow together, to develop poise and symmetry.

Double Yoga celebrates life. The teachings of Yoga urge you to live fully, to experience inner beauty and appreciate the beauty in others, and to free yourself from the bondage of routine. Life can be an adventure of constant learning, of caring and sharing without authority, and of enlightenment born in the joy of spontaneous unfolding.

Many people come to Yoga for its physical benefits and discover themselves in the process. Is it possible to approach Hatha Yoga only on the physical level? Can the physical be divided from the mental? Yoga teaches that body and mind exist on the same continuum. The law that declares energy and matter to be interchangeable underlines this Yogic concept of the basic unity of mind and body. Study of the body leads to the same source as the exploration of space, science, or mystic truth.

As you learn to appreciate the strength, grace, and mystery of the human being, you will become sensitive to the beauty of nature, the earth, the stars. As you experience the body's wholeness and intelligence, the illusion of separateness will begin to dissolve and you will feel your oneness with the universe. Then perhaps in the silence of a moment, in the joy of stillness, you may perceive something (a no-thing) that is beyond thought, explanation, and words, that is indescribable—the essence of Yoga, of life.

G.W.

The Ten Systems

The body is a miraculous machine, the result of millions of years of evolution. We take it for granted and rarely observe what a marvel it is. Too often we abuse our bodies and cause premature aging and dullness. What is aging? The body will wear out in time, even though it is capable of self-repair and healing. Yet, through correct care and use, the body will become stronger, more alert and energetic, and remain so well into old age. Health is the natural state, disease the sign of imbalance and wrong living. Hatha Yoga teaches us how to live wholly and maintain the body at its peak.

The body degenerates as a result of wrong living and aging. This process includes stiffening, immobility, poor circulation, and toxicity. Hatha Yoga restores flexibility and mobility. It improves circulation, nerve and gland efficiency, stamina, and breathing capacity. Hatha Yoga relieves stress, increases energy and vitality, and improves digestion, assimilation, and elimination. As you break through physical barriers, you will find mental barriers dissolving as well. Your mind will become more alert, calm, efficient, and open. If you are young, you will reach new levels of awareness as your physical abilities increase. Your youth will be prolonged. If you are older, you will regain the vitality, energy, and suppleness of youth. No matter what your age, you will experience a sense of peace, beauty, and joy that cannot be explained in words.

Hatha Yoga puts the responsibility for health and the means for attaining it into your own hands. The body is an interrelationship of ten equally vital systems. The practice of Yoga *asanas* (*aah*-sun-ahs, poses) ensures the healthy, balanced functioning of these ten systems.

1. *The Skeletal System:* Science has shown that even the bones increase in strength through use. Full mobility requires free movement of all the joints. The *asanas* move each joint to its limit every day. You are able to maintain your present mobility while slowly improving beyond your current range of movement.

2. *The Muscular System:* Efficient muscles are long, free of stored tensions, and possess good tone. The mental stress stored in the muscles is removed through practice of the poses. Longer muscles use less energy than shorter ones for the same task. When every muscle is stretched to

capacity each day, the accumulated tension, tightness, and shortening are counteracted and the body retains its suppleness.

3. *The Circulatory System:* The heart begins beating during the fourth week after conception. Though an adult's heart weighs less than a pound, it pumps 2,000 gallons of blood each day (50 million gallons over a lifetime) through 100,000 miles of blood vessels! The Yogic poses increase the flow of blood to specific areas of the body so that all parts are nourished in turn.

4. *The Nervous System:* Most of the body's nerves connect to the brain through the spinal cord. Pressure on the nerves can result in numerous physical problems. The *asanas* keep the spine flexible so there is no impingement on the nerves. Blood and energy are directed to specific nerve plexi in various poses.

5. *The Digestive System:* Proper care of the digestive system, which also implies eating intelligently, is an important part of Yoga. Certain poses stimulate the digestive system, relieve pressure on nerves associated with digestion, alleviate internal congestion, and promote good assimilation.

6. *The Eliminative System:* Getting wastes out of the body is as important as getting nutrients in. Yogic techniques cleanse the intestinal tract, stimulate peristalsis, cleanse the kidneys and skin, and promote proper elimination.

7. *The Respiratory System:* Oxygen is the element most used by the body. Incomplete respiration will impair every other bodily function. The lungs serve not only to bring in oxygen but also to eliminate carbon dioxide and other waste gases. Senility, poor concentration, and mental fatigue can be caused by lack of oxygen in the brain cells. Deep breathing in the poses cleanses the lungs and stimulates the cardiovascular system. Breath is the life-force and is directly related to vitality and mental balance. The Yogi develops a strong respiratory system, a strong breath, a powerful life-force.

8. *The Endocrine System:* The glands regulate the body's metabolism and vital functions, including energy level, demeanor, mental state, and sexual drive. The tonic poses have a balanc-

ing effect. Certain poses balance specific glands, such as the pituitary and pineal in the Head Stand and the thyroid and parathyroid in the Shoulder Stand.

9. *The Pranic System: Prana* is the life-force and the basis of Yoga practices. We have all felt this energy, knowingly or unknowingly, in the presence of a powerful person, in a healing moment, or after suffering an injury, when we instinctively clasp the wound and breathe deeply. *Prana* is our connection to the cosmos and source of life. We may feel independent, but at least 21,600 times a day the ebb and flow of our breath reminds us of our cosmic connection. Yogis meditate on the sound of the breath. Through Yogic breathing and poses one can have a direct experience of this energy and connect with its abundance.

10. *The Mental System:* A sound mind requires a sound body. The correct practice of Yoga produces mental clarity and a quality of attention that pervades the whole body. To achieve mental wholeness, we must understand the nature of thought and its role in daily life and in right action. This understanding is the fruit of self-observation and inquiry, the purpose of Yoga.

The Principles of Yoga

Start Where You Are

The only place to begin is exactly where you are. Yoga views competition and comparison as a useless waste of energy. It considers the joy of excellence in action a higher source of energy than competition. Certainly you may check yourself against a more advanced person in order to learn, but to measure yourself against another and conclude you are inferior or superior is counter-productive. Ignore the Western imperative to compete and rank yourself. Don't let your idea of your physical limitations stop you from beginning. You will probably discover that your mental images of what you can and cannot do are more limiting than your body's abilities. In Yoga the intention is to learn from moment to moment. What you were incapable of yesterday may be possible today, and perhaps what you were able to do yesterday is not possible today. Therefore be attentive each moment. There is a great saying: "Start where you are and stay there."
It doesn't imply stagnation, for there will be constant change and growth. It means having the wisdom to make the most of the present.

About Time

Learning the basics of Hatha Yoga need not take long. How long depends on how seriously you practice and your physical state when you begin. There is no state one attains called "now I have learned, now I am finished." Since the body is constantly changing, learning Yoga can be a lifelong experience. The essence of Yoga is outside the framework of time in which we are caught and bound. Practice Yoga without being conscious of time, with complete attention to the moment. Then Yoga will become a continuous learning process, joyfully unfolding and evolving.

Breathing

Life-force is called *prana (prah*-nah). The system of Hatha Yoga *asanas* and breathing is based on balancing and increasing the flow of *prana* in the body. *Prana* exists in all things and is abundant in air, sunlight, food, and water. We can experience *prana* as a movement of energy in the body, in the touch of another, and as a magnetic, radiant presence. Breathing is the key to understanding *prana* and energy. One who has strong lungs and good breathing capacity usually has abundant energy. Breathing is also influenced by one's mental state. When the mind is clear and balanced, the breath is even and rhythmic. When the mind is nervous and tense, the breath is strained and erratic. Watch for these things in your practice and keep your breath flowing smoothly.

During the practice of Yoga breathe only through the nostrils, not through the mouth. The nasal passages filter and warm the air, preparing it for the lungs. There is an energy network that corresponds to the nervous system called *nadis (nah*-dees). Where there are nerves, there are *nadis*. Energy is absorbed and flows through these *nadis*. The nasal passages have more nerve endings than the mouth, and consequently more *prana* is absorbed during nasal breathing, which also has a balancing effect on the nervous system. And that is what the nose is for— breathing! Stop reading for a moment and with your eyes closed take a few deep breaths in and out through the nose. Then take a few breaths in and out through the mouth. You will immediately notice the difference. Always breathe through the nose unless your nasal passages are clogged.

When learning a new pose and concentrating, one tends to hold the breath. Notice if you do this and keep the breath moving. When holding the poses, breathe evenly, smoothly, and deeply. Inhaling increases strength and firmness in the muscles. Exhaling relaxes and softens them. Therefore when twisting or stretching into a position, exhale slowly to make the muscles and the body pliable. This will prevent strain and allow you to go further into the pose.

Make sure you are able to breathe properly and to fill the lungs completely. Lie on your back and begin inhaling and exhaling slowly. First become aware of correct diaphragmatic breathing. As you inhale, the downward movement of the diaphragm should push your stomach outward. As you exhale, the stomach will sink back down. This correct breathing feels almost like the stomach is moving the air or is actually filling with air. The next step is to learn to fill the lungs completely. When inhaling, bring the air into the bottom of the lungs with the diaphragm. Then continue inhaling to open and expand the rib cage upward *and* out to the sides. Exhale simultaneously with the chest and stomach (diaphragm). After you practice this awhile on your back, and this breathing begins to feel natural, try it in a sitting position. Learn to breathe smoothly and evenly, and avoid breathing solely with the chest.

There is a special breathing technique called *ujaayi* (ōō-*jaah*-yee) that can be used to keep your attention, energy level, and mind steady during the practice of Hatha Yoga. In *ujaayi* the glottis is kept partially closed during inhalation and exhalation. You may learn this technique from a teacher or through the following exercise: Whisper the word *purrrrrr,* holding the *rrrrrr* a few seconds. Now whisper *purrrrr* on both the inhalation and exhalation. Don't make the sound too loud and keep it smooth and even. When you are able to whisper this sound through the mouth evenly in and out, close your mouth and continue the sound through the nostrils on inhalation and exhalation. Keep the throat relaxed. This is *ujaayi.*

Concentration and Attention

Concentration is the focusing of awareness on a single point. Concentration is necessary in learning poses, for the mind must check many points and make adjustments and corrections. Eventually, as you learn a pose thoroughly, concentration ends and attention comes into being. In attention you are totally aware of the entire body without focusing. Attention cannot be practiced or cultivated—it simply happens. Any forcing or effort toward it immediately results in concentration. Notice the difference and notice the process in yourself. Let attention happen.

Symmetry and Balance

Correctly practiced, Yoga brings the body into equilibrium and alignment. The skeleton is supported by the muscular system and uneven development of the muscles or stored-up tension can throw off the body's alignment. In our daily activities, including moving, sitting, and lying down, we have developed patterns and habits. We bend in a certain way, sit, stand, and sleep in patterned ways, and create imbalances in our bodily structure. Over the years this can cause poor posture, stiffness, pain, tension, and uneven wear on joints and discs. During the practice of Yoga poses the tense, stiff muscle sets and joints quickly become apparent. The poses and complementary counterposes are symmetrical and realign the body. The new alignment that develops in the practice of Yoga will eventually become natural so that you carry yourself properly and have better posture in daily life. When doing Double Yoga try to overcome any imbalance and unevenness you discover in your body. Do some extra work on your weak or stiff areas. We may be conditioned to believe we are right- or left-handed and -sided, yet both sides of the body can be developed relatively equally. Don't be one-sided—good advice for Yoga and for life. Develop symmetry and balance, grace and beauty.

Work Versus Strain

To keep the musculature healthy and toned, regular activity is necessary. Even the bones become stronger through use. Working your muscles beyond their usual level of activity is what signals them to increase in strength. Don't confuse the Yogic principle of not straining with not working. Strain is a tense pushing beyond your proper limit. Straining in the poses may cause injury. Working intelligently in the poses will energize and strengthen your body.

The Body's Intelligence

An important principle in Hatha Yoga is learning to listen to your body's intelligence. The body does not speak in words but it communicates loudly and clearly if you listen. It will teach you correct movement and point out mistakes, singing when you work and asking for rest, too. Pain is one of the voices of the body. Sharp pains tell you to stop, dull pains to breathe and go slowly, for you are moving energy into new areas. This intelligence, this life-force in your body, is a great teacher. Listen to it.

Strength and Flexibility

Hatha Yoga is the Yoga of sun *(ha)* and moon *(tha)*. The sun symbolizes strength, heating, and expansion; the moon, flexibility, cooling, and contraction. Harmonizing and balancing these energies is one purpose of Hatha Yoga. Strength without flexibility causes rigidity and flexibility without strength leads to fragility. Both sun and moon energies are combined in each pose. Don't do the poses rigidly (too much *ha)* or limply (too much *tha)*. Stretch into each position and hold it dynamically.

Extending the Spine

Yoga considers the spine to be a continuation of the brain. Most of the nerves in the body pass through and are protected by the spine. Yogis measure aging by the condition of the spine. As one gets older, it becomes more rigid, affecting both body and mind. A supple spine is essential for maintaining vitality, health, and youth. Gravity constantly pulls the body down so that the muscles supporting the vertebrae must work to keep the spine from collapsing. The Yogic poses stretch and extend the spinal column, increasing the space between vertebrae. Be sure to keep your back extended whenever you twist or bend forward or backward. Don't let your back shorten or collapse in any pose.

Attunement

Double Yoga requires attunement to your partner. When one partner pushes too much or doesn't support enough, both will slip. As in any close relationship, each Yoga partner will mirror the other's mistakes and imbalances. Both must develop verbal and nonverbal communication, sensitivity, patience, and trust and each must be aware of the effects of one another's movements. First there are two people and two poses meshing together. Then, as attunement develops, the double pose is transformed into one pose—a dynamic interaction of energy.

Yoga and Athletics

Sports and athletic activities are not incompatible with Yoga. On the contrary, the two complement each other quite well, with Yoga often increasing athletic performance. Most sports cause taut muscles and create imbalances because of the uneven use of muscle groups or one side of the body. This pulls the skeleton out of alignment. Yoga is invaluable for correcting these defects. Certain activities—weight lifting and running, for example—can cause severe shortening of the muscles. When this happens, it is advisable to curtail the activity until flexibility and balance are restored with Yoga. The stretching of Yoga *asanas* produces longer muscles, and longer muscles use energy more efficiently and are less prone to injury. For all these reasons, and because it improves coordination, alertness, efficiency, and whole-body use, Yoga poses are excellent training for the athlete.

Movement of Energy

Yoga recognizes the existence of an energy body that animates and energizes the physical body. This energy body is charged and vitalized through the practice of Yogic poses. That is why it's important to learn to hold the poses dynamically. Don't allow awareness to become dulled. Keep the energy flowing, the body alive and radiant. Even when your physical body cannot move all the way into a pose, you will be able to feel the correct position and action by moving your energy body properly. For example, when the instructions call for extending or twisting the spine and you cannot do the movement fully, feel your energy body extending or twisting into the position. Eventually your physical body will follow.

The Threshold

Always stay on the threshold of your ability. Each body has its own threshold, which changes from day to day. Even an advanced student accumulates tightness and imbalances because modern life is governed by psychological stresses and physical inactivity—sitting, driving, standing for long periods. Each day we must discover our thresholds, which are defined by the limits of flexibility and strength and are signaled by pain or immobility. As you approach your limit, your body will begin signaling you with mild pain. Don't force, stay just in back of the pain or move and breathe gently into it. Yoga is a living science, a continuous learning. We too easily seek the comfort of getting to a place where we can go back to sleep. In Yoga one learns to stay on the threshold and penetrate the unknown.

Loving and Leaving the Body

Our bodies are the most basic requirement for action in this world. Hatha Yoga points out the need to care for and maintain the body. How would you act if someone gave you an automobile and told you that this would be the only car you would ever own throughout your life? How would you maintain this auto? Would you use poor-quality gas and oil? Or would you treat your auto with great care and attention, knowing it must last your entire life? We have only one body to get us through life. If we abuse and destroy our body, it will become a burden. Of course, the body will eventually wear out no matter how well we care for it. That is why Hatha Yoga teaches that bodily attachment and vanity bring pain and suffering. Yoga confronts us with this paradox: Love and care for the body, but don't become so attached to it that you forget it is ephemeral.

Relaxation

Relaxation has nearly become a lost art in our high-speed society. Physical tension affects the mind, just as a nervous, tense, or chattering mind affects the body. Each one reflects and becomes the other. Total relaxation cannot be achieved by simply resting or engaging in some diversion. Real relaxation—rejuvenation and renewal—is a positive state of balance and equilibrium in the body and mind and is attained through action. Hatha Yoga allows you to release pent-up energies, stored tensions, and energy blocks. It restores you to wholeness and makes it possible to experience real relaxation and equanimity.

When you are first learning the poses, you may tire quickly. This is easily overcome through regular practice and by slowly increasing the time spent in the poses as your abilities improve. In the beginning, rest a little between poses, but not too long or the body will cool and lose energy. As you progress, you will find that you no longer need to rest between poses.

End each session with a period of conscious rest. Lie quietly but use your mind to bring about the full effect. As you lie on your back, consciously relax your entire body, letting your weight rest completely on the floor. Release any tightness or tension and allow your body to become soft. Take a few deep breaths, then let the breathing become slow and quiet. If you rest completely in this way for five to fifteen minutes, you will experience well-being.

General Instructions

1. Practice in an environment that is clean, orderly, and free of distractions. Don't practice in the hot sun.

2. It is best to do the Standing Poses on a hard, nonslip, level surface. The other poses—Assisting, Back Bend, Inverted, Forward Bend, Sitting, and Twists—may be practiced on a blanket, mat, or carpet.

3. Generally the postures should be held for thirty seconds to one minute. Forward bends and inverted poses are held for two to five minutes. Gradually increase the period of time you hold a pose. Advanced students may hold for longer times and repeat more.

4. Don't hold a pose beyond your ability to come out of it with control.

5. Always practice attentively. Don't do the poses half consciously or mechanically. Be attentive to the position of all bodily parts, the correct movements, breathing, proper alignment, and symmetry.

6. The manner in which you move into and out of each pose is part of the pose. Avoid clumsy, jerked movements. As you progress, your movements should become smoother and more graceful until you can flow from one pose to another.

7. When holding a position with your partner, if you feel the energy exchange and flow begin to diminish, change the pose or rest.

8. You may not always have a partner available. The general instructions and many of the photographs can be used to exercise alone, which is valuable; you are encouraged to keep your practice regular.

9. Some soreness is normal when the muscles are being toned and strengthened to new limits and when new sets of muscles are being used. This can be relieved by a hot bath, some stretching, or a massage with a deep-heating rub. The best treatment, however, is regular practice. If you have any medical problems or have not done any regular exercise for a long time, you should check with your doctor before you begin a program of Yoga. Most people can do Yoga safely. It is a balanced exercise that has been found to be beneficial for people of all ages and body conditions.

10. Yoga in the morning dissipates sluggishness, improves mobility, and gets the circulation going. Morning Yoga makes one alert so that the whole day goes better. Evening Yoga relaxes and removes the tensions and imbalances accumulated during the day.

11. On cold mornings a hot shower or bath will make doing the poses easier.

12. The poses should be done on an empty stomach.

13. If in any of the positions you are unable to reach and clasp a hand or foot as called for in the instructions, use a belt loop to span the gap.

14. You and your partner may not be able to match yourselves exactly to the positions shown in the photographs. Make suitable adjustments according to your relative sizes and flexibilities.

15. Doing the poses in front of a mirror occasionally is valuable for checking symmetry and alignment. If possible, install a full-length mirror in the room where you practice.

16. You may find the poses easier to learn if a friend reads the instructions to you as you assume the positions. Or you may want to dictate the instructions into a tape recorder and play them back as you practice.

17. In poses where you must change to do the left and right sides, the instructions are given for only one side to avoid confusion. To change sides, simply reverse the position or follow the directions again from the beginning on the other side.

18. Be sure not to strain the face or tense the neck in any pose (the neck is a major site of stored tension). When holding a pose, check if you have a tendency to tighten your face or neck. Once you are aware of this tightening habit, you will be able to end it and keep the energy moving throughout your body. Then even during the day you will prevent this accumulation of tension.

19. After learning the basics of Double Yoga and acquiring a feel for the system, create your own double poses to suit your bodies and abilities.

20. The poses vary from easy ones for beginners to more difficult ones, designated by ☀, for advanced students. You may be able to do many of the poses labeled difficult, but build up to them gradually, listening to the limits of your body. Choose some poses from each group:

Standing Poses, Forward Bends, Back Bends, Inverted Poses, Twists, and Sitting Poses. In that way you will derive full benefit by exercising all areas of the body and all muscles and joints. Consult the section on Suggested Practice Sessions for guidance.

21. Mechanical, robotlike action will not be possible if you are attentive in your practice. Once you have learned the basics of a pose, you can begin the real exploration. You will never get bored.

22. Always hold the poses as correctly as your ability allows, using the instructions and photographs as a guide. Incorrect holding will only reinforce bad habits and prevent you from overcoming weaknesses. It is better to hold a pose for a shorter period of time in a correct position than for the suggested time, or longer, incorrectly.

23. As you progress in ability and understanding, reread The Principles of Yoga, the Detail Instructions, and these General Instructions from time to time. Once you have gained experience, you will have a different perspective and be better able to absorb details. Above all, have fun!

Detail Photographs and Instructions

These detail photographs and instructions explain specific movements done in the poses that make a big difference in the correctness and quality of a position. Study these and incorporate the movements into your practice.

Foot Alignment

In many standing positions the instructions call for aligning the heel and toe of the front facing foot with the arch of the rear foot. Standing on a line on the floor makes this easy to learn. Photo 1 shows the correct position with the front foot on the line and the rear foot across the line and slightly turned in.

FOOT POSITION

INCORRECT: In standing poses the feet should always be pressed evenly into the floor. The incorrect position in Photo 2 shows the foot rolled in and down into the direction of the posture.

CORRECT: In Photo 3 the foot presses evenly on both sides. This creates a lift in the foot and strengthens the arch and ankle. In the correct position more energy moves up the

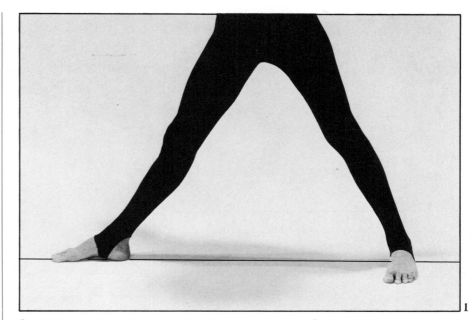

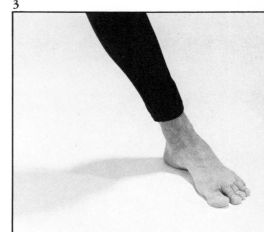

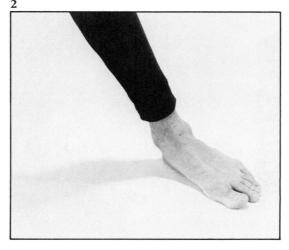

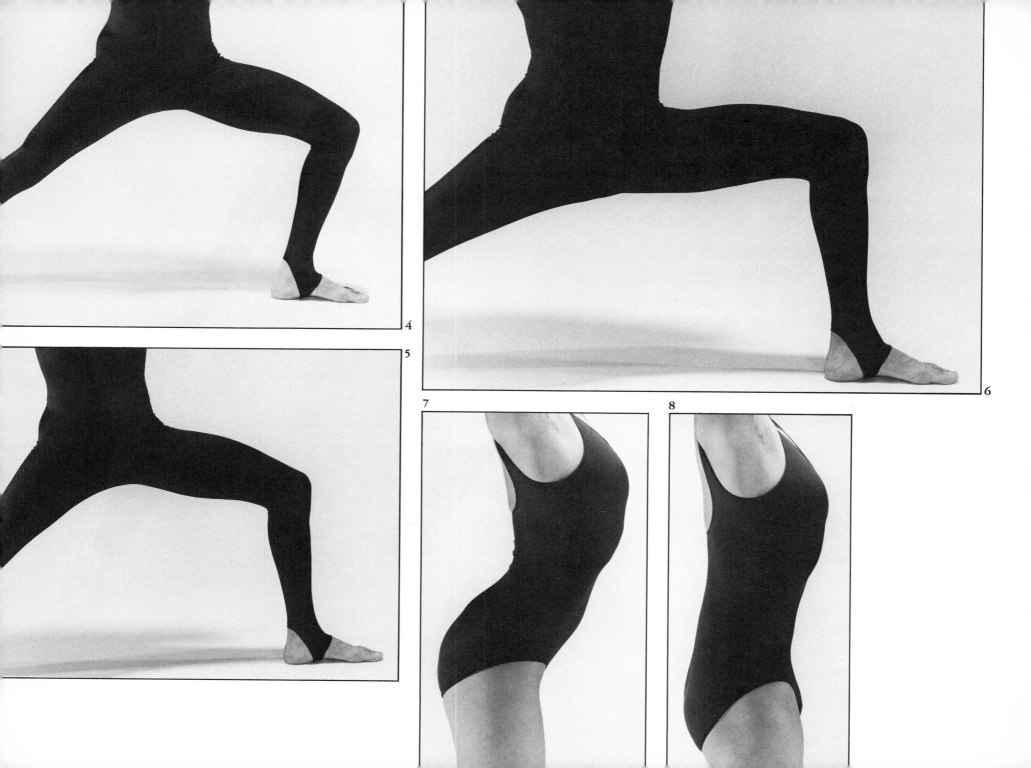

4

5

6

7

8

leg, energizing the whole pose. When the foot is in the rear in a standing posture, press the outside edge even more firmly to get the proper lift in the arch and inner ankle.

Right-Angle Knee Movements

INCORRECT: The knee is overextended in Photo 4, at less than a right angle. Right-angle poses should not be done in this way, for the incorrect movement can strain the knee. The shinbone must always be kept vertical when holding right-angle poses.

ACCEPTABLE: In Photo 5 the thigh has not been brought down to form a right angle, but the shinbone is almost vertical and the knee is over the ankle. This position is useful for beginners and people with weak or injured knees. It can help strengthen the knees and thighs when a full right-angle position is too much of a strain.

CORRECT: Photo 6 shows the correct, full right-angle position. Notice that the shinbone is vertical and perpendicular to the thigh and the floor. The thigh is parallel to the floor and at a right angle to the torso.

Tucking the Tailbone

INCORRECT: The instructions for poses often state, "Tuck the tailbone down." In Photo 7 the tailbone and hips are protruding, causing the back to sway. This incorrect movement can cause lumbar pain in back bends and prevent the flow of energy up the body in standing poses. There is compression in the lower back and the spine isn't properly elongated.

CORRECT: Photo 8 shows the correct movement. The tailbone is tucked down. The pelvis is open, the spine is long, and energy can now flow. In back bends the weight of the body will be evenly distributed along the legs and spine.

Extending Both Sides of the Torso

INCORRECT: When bending or twisting from the hips, both sides of the torso should work and be kept parallel. In Photo 9, showing the Triangle, the lower side of the torso is compressing and not working. This cuts off circulation and causes these muscles to bunch up rather than stretch.

CORRECT: In Photo 10 the lower side of the torso is parallel to the upper and is working a little harder to extend into the bend. This correct movement feels more dynamic and strengthens the back.

Raising the Rib Cage and Extending Upward

INCORRECT: In many poses the arms are held overhead or the instructions call for extending them upward. In Photo 11, though the arms and shoulders are raised, the movement is coming only from the shoulders and there is no life in the pose. The body is sagging and looks out of shape.

CORRECT: The lift of the arms and shoulders in Photo 12 is coming all the way from the legs. The rib cage is also extending up and there is an almost visible flow of energy upward. The whole body looks different, it comes alive.

Extending the Spine

INCORRECT: The incorrect position, Photo 13, looks lifeless. The stomach and upper spine are compressed and tense, so little energy can flow between the back and legs.

CORRECT: The correct movement, Photo 14, is to extend forward, making both sides of the spine equal in length. There is pull from the top of the head to the legs, and there is vitality in the pose. Extending the spine in this way in forward bends and twists not only lengthens the muscles but tones them as well. Energy flows through all parts of the body and the nervous system is rejuvenated. When the instructions say to extend the spine or flatten the back, this is the movement referred to.

9

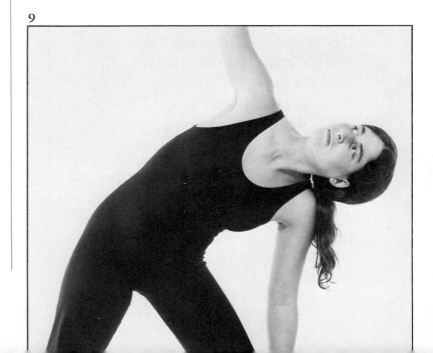

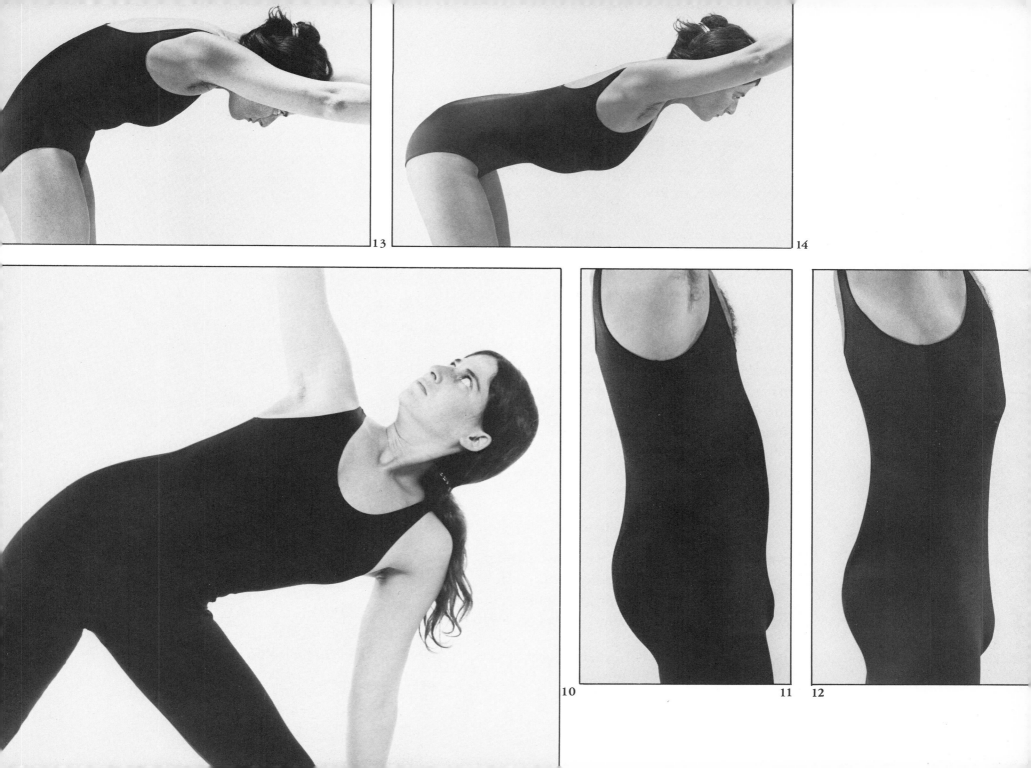

13

14

10

11

12

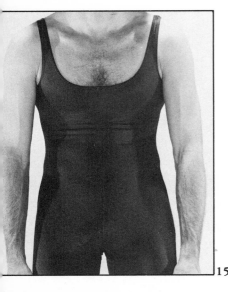

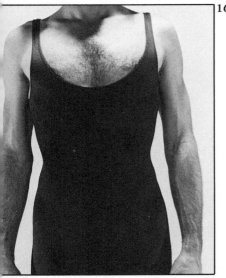

15

16

Lifting and Expanding the Chest

INCORRECT: The chest is not open and looks almost sunken in Photo 15. The chest is a major seat of energy in the body. People with great energy usually have broad chests that can open and expand to fill the lungs deeply with air. A very important goal of Hatha Yoga is to free the intercostal muscles and open the chest to increase your energy level.

CORRECT: Photo 16 shows the chest expanded, open, and lifted so that the shoulders naturally roll back. This is done without arching the spine. The body looks younger and more radiant. When the instructions say to lift and open the chest, this is the movement referred to.

Neck Extension

INCORRECT: Since many nerves pass through the neck, it is a storage area for tension. In Photo 17 the neck is compressed, which constricts the flow of energy and creates tension.

CORRECT: The neck is lifted and extended in Photo 18. The muscles are long and soft, energy can flow freely, and the neck looks relaxed. Releasing tension in the neck to increase mobility and the flow of nerve energy is one of the great benefits of Hatha Yoga.

Neck Rotation

INCORRECT: In Photo 19 the neck is not only compressed but bent back as it was turned. Again, this prevents the flow of energy and can cause tension or cramps in the neck.

CORRECT: The correct movement when turning the head in Yogic poses, shown in Photo 20, is to extend the neck and rotate it on the same plane. This keeps the cervical area long, increases space between the vertebrae internally and from the head to the shoulder externally; this ensures the flow of energy.

Hand Position

INCORRECT: The hand in Photo 21 is compressed and tense. Another common error is a limp, inactive hand with no energy.

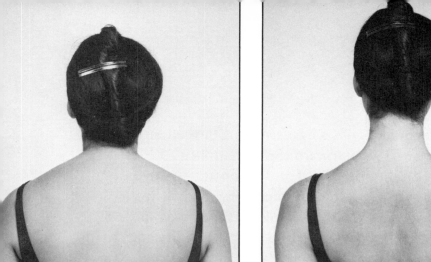

17

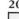

18

19

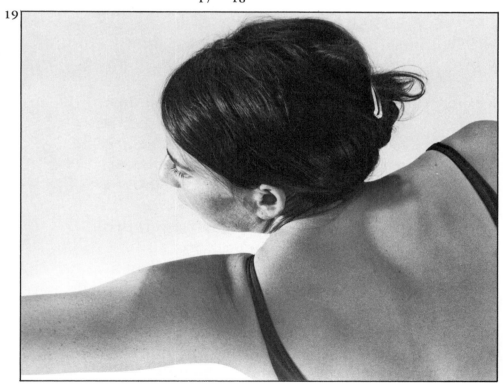

20

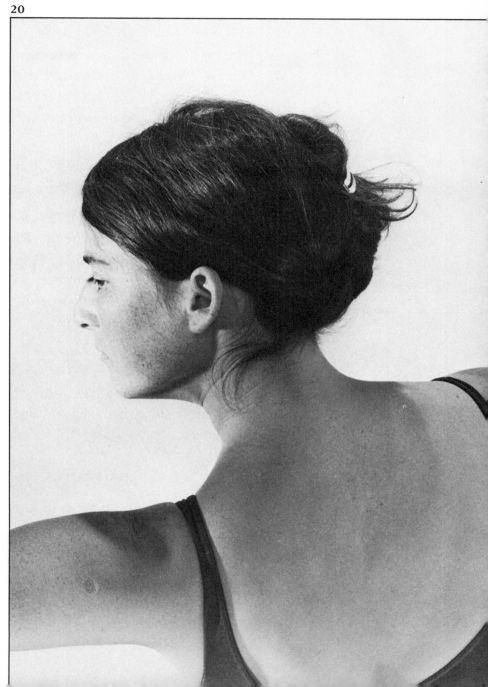

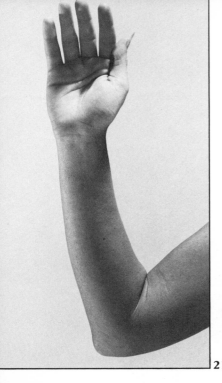

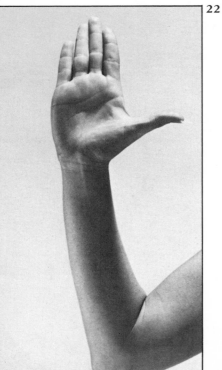

21

22

CORRECT: In the correct position of Photo 22 the palm is opened fully and the thumb is spread to the side. This stretches the hand and finger muscles and increases energy flow along the arm.

Cross-Legged Positions

Many Yogic poses are done in a sitting position. The Lotus pose is the most famous and is very stable, but most sitting positions can also be done in a simpler variation. Any one of the following can be substituted for the Lotus position shown in later poses.

CROSS-LEGGED

This is the easiest position, shown in Photo 23. Simply sit with the legs folded, feet under the knees.

HALF LOTUS

Fold one leg in and place it under the other thigh, as in Photo 24. Fold the other leg in and place it on top of the opposite thigh. Bring the knees close enough together so that the ankle is not contorted. One of the best ways to work toward the more difficult Lotus is to sit in the Half Lotus whenever possible during the day. Your knees may not touch the floor at first, but by regular practice the hip joints and quadriceps will gain flexibility and you will be able to place your knees on the floor. Be sure to alternate legs so both are stretched equally.

LOTUS

Sit with the legs extended and pull one foot high onto the opposite thigh, Photo 25. Then fold the other leg, pulling the foot onto the top of the opposite thigh, Photo 26. *Do not force the knees.* If you cannot assume this position easily, wait until you acquire more flexibility. Sitting in the Cross-Legged or Half Lotus pose, and regular practice of Hatha Yoga, will prepare you for the full Lotus. It is a wonderful position, worth working up to, for it creates mobility in the ankles, knees, and hips. You will find that when you sit in the Lotus, energy flows through your entire body and your brain becomes more alert.

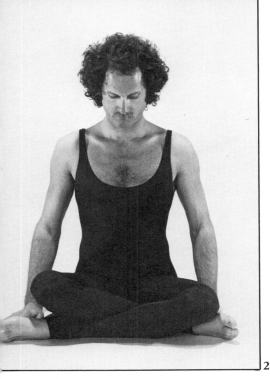

23

24

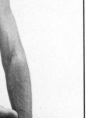

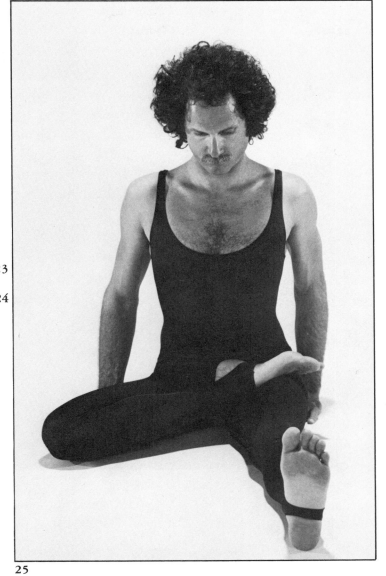

25

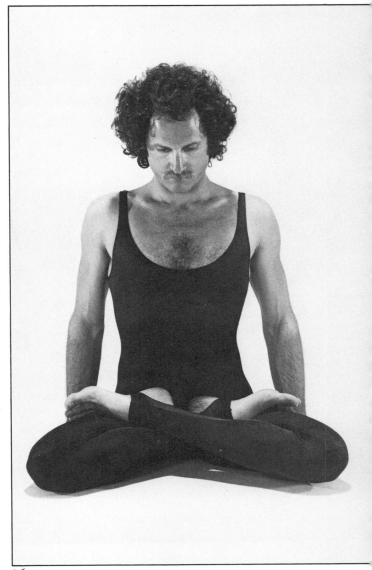

26

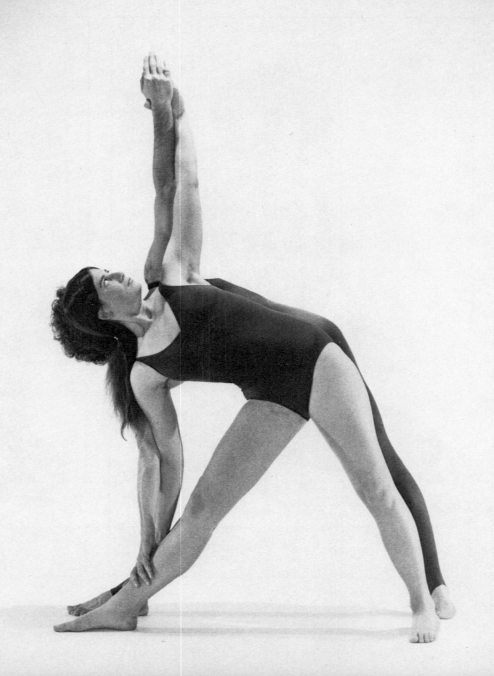

THE TRIANGLE

Stand back to back against your partner and spread your legs three feet apart. If you are of different heights, keep your front feet even and make the necessary adjustment with your rear feet. Holding hands, raise your arms out to the side at shoulder level, keeping them parallel to the floor. Then turn one foot out and the other slightly in, keeping the center of the forward heel and toe in line with the rear arch as shown. This is the basic foot position in many standing poses (see Photo 1). In the Triangle one partner does a mirror image on the opposite side. Now, exhaling, extend the leading arm and torso out over the forward leg and reach down to grasp your partner's right ankle (or higher on the leg, according to flexibility). Stretch up with the opposite arm and turn your head toward the ceiling. Notice that your arms cross and each partner's arm is supported on the other partner's leg. Use this double posture to increase your extension. Make sure your shoulders and spines are evenly pressed together. To improve the pose, work to keep the torso straight so that the bend comes from the hips, not the ribs. Knees should be straight and the tailbone tucked down. Do not turn the hips, but keep them facing forward. After holding, extend up, change legs, and repeat on the other side.

BENEFITS: Just as the triangle is the most basic geometric structure in nature, the Triangle pose is the building block of other positions in Yoga. Take the time to learn it correctly and then apply its principles to the other poses. The Triangle tones all the muscles, especially those in the legs. To do it properly, you must become attentive to your whole body simultaneously.

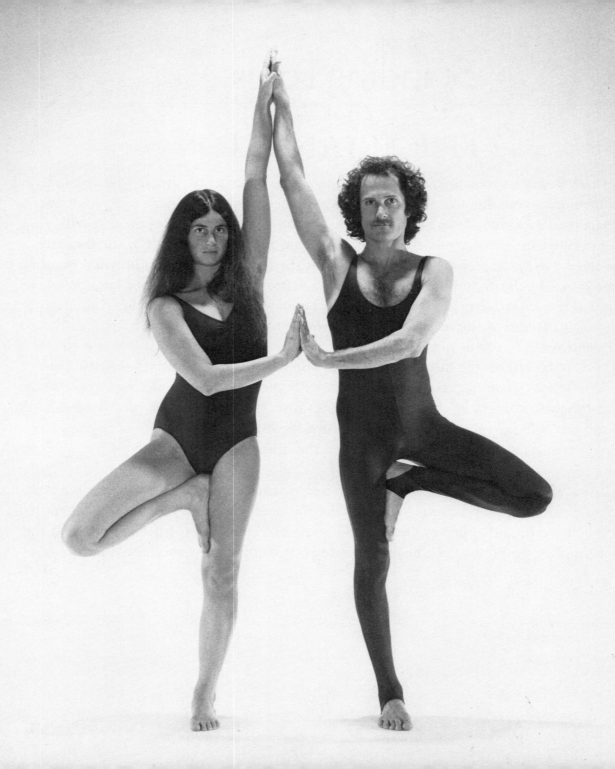

THE TREE I

Stand about two feet apart with your feet parallel. Raise your inside arm and clasp your partner's hand while lifting your outside foot as high as possible onto your inner thigh. Lock the inside leg, stand erect, and touch your partner's hand lightly with your free hand. Do not lean on each other. Stand straight, keep the chest lifted, tailbone tucked down, hips even. Remain as still as possible, breathing smoothly and gazing at one spot. Hold, extending up into the pose, then repeat on the other side.

BENEFITS: Though an easy pose, the Tree I demands firm balance, or you will knock your partner over. It strengthens the ankles and legs and teaches attentive stillness.

THE TREE II

Stand shoulder to shoulder with your partner, your feet about twelve inches apart and parallel. Simultaneously lift your outer legs high to the front of the thigh and clasp each other's foot with your inside arm. Reach up and touch hands. Stand straight and breathe evenly. Hold, extending up into the pose, then repeat on the other side.

BENEFITS: This pose stretches the thighs, increases knee flexibility, and improves balance.

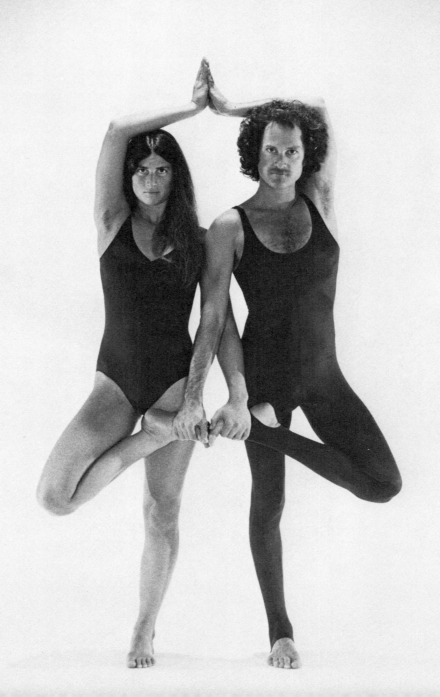

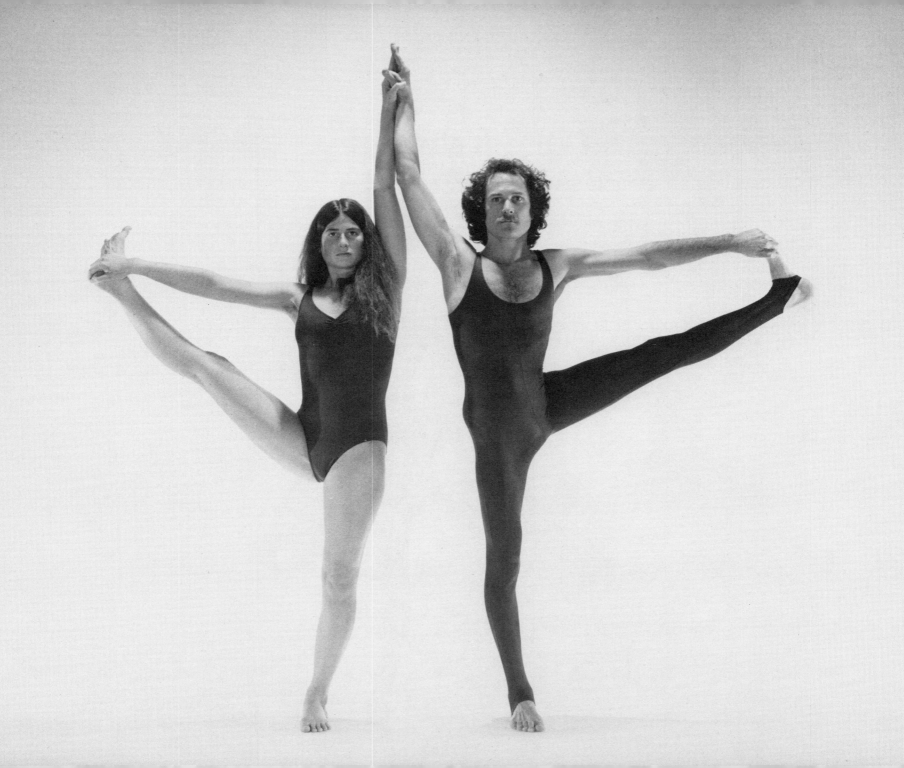

THE BIG TOE

Stand two to three feet apart, extend your arms up, and hold hands. Bend the outside leg and hold the big toe firmly with the hand or fingers (or you may grasp the heel). Then straighten the leg, extending it out to the side. Stretch up and lift the chest, being careful to lock both knees and tuck the tailbone down to make the spine straight. If you cannot straighten your raised leg, loop a belt or rope over the arch of your foot and grab the belt. Hold, then repeat on the other side.

BENEFITS: This pose stretches and strengthens the muscles of the inner legs and increases hip joint flexibility. It also improves balance and concentration.

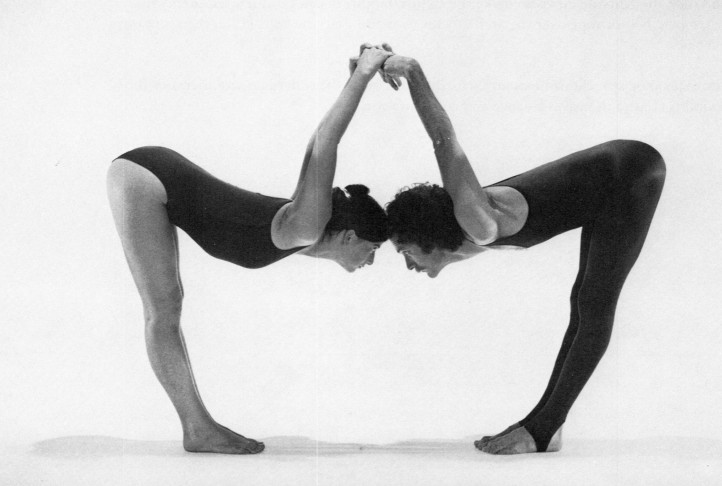

THE ROYAL CROWN

Stand about three feet apart so that your foreheads touch when you bend forward. Clasp your hands behind your back, inhale, and lift your chest. Then bend forward, exhaling, keeping your back straight and bringing your arms over your head to meet and hold your partner's hands. Touch foreheads, breathing smoothly, and look into each other's eyes. The effects of this pose can be increased by pressing foreheads and then pushing away to extend the spine while lifting with the arms.

BENEFITS: This pose stretches your body from the back of your legs all the way to the top of your spine, relieving tension. It strengthens the back and loosens the shoulders.

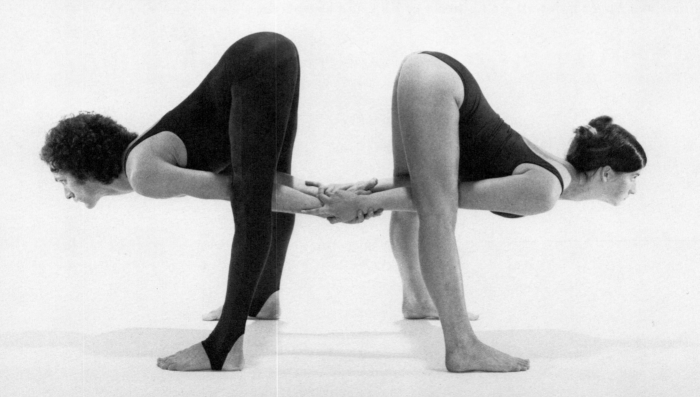

THE PUMP

Stand back to back about two feet from your partner with your legs three feet apart. Bend forward, reaching through your legs to grab your partner's wrists. Stretch your torso forward, arching it slightly according to your flexibility, and stretch the backs of your legs. Hold for thirty seconds, then begin a slow pumplike motion in which one partner arches up, pulling the other through the legs, and then the other arches up, pulling the first partner down. Inhale as you arch up and exhale as you are pulled down.

BENEFITS: The spread of the legs and arching of the torso required by this pose give a unique stretch to the backs of the legs, hips, inner legs, and spine. The pumping motion warms up and strengthens these areas very quickly. Clasping the wrists of your partner allows you to stretch the muscles intensely.

THE FENCE

Stand about two feet apart. Each partner balances on the outer leg while lifting the inner leg, one in front and one behind. Grab your partner's heel or ankle and shoulders as shown. Extend up straight, face forward, keeping your feet parallel and raised ankles flexed back. Like a well-built fence, this pose creates many right angles. Hold, breathing evenly and gazing at a point, then repeat on the other side.

BENEFITS: The inner thighs and hip joints are stretched, the legs and ankles are strengthened, and balance is improved.

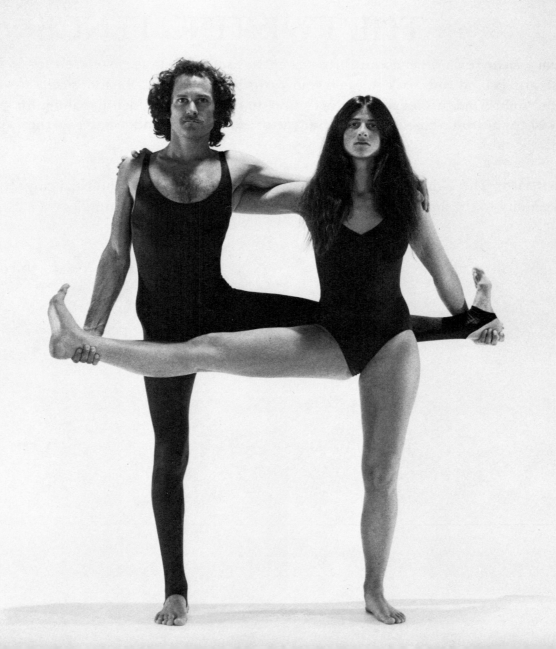

THE TWISTING FENCE

Stand facing each other about three feet apart. Each of you raises your left leg and reaches your left arm behind your back to catch your partner's ankle. Press the foot firmly to your hip. Place your right hand behind your partner's neck to the right shoulder. Exhaling, lift your chest and twist toward your raised leg. Use your partner for leverage and to increase the twist. Hold, then change sides.

BENEFITS: The Twisting Fence provides the benefits of twisting and balancing. It gives lateral flexibility to the hips and spine while stretching the outer thigh muscles.

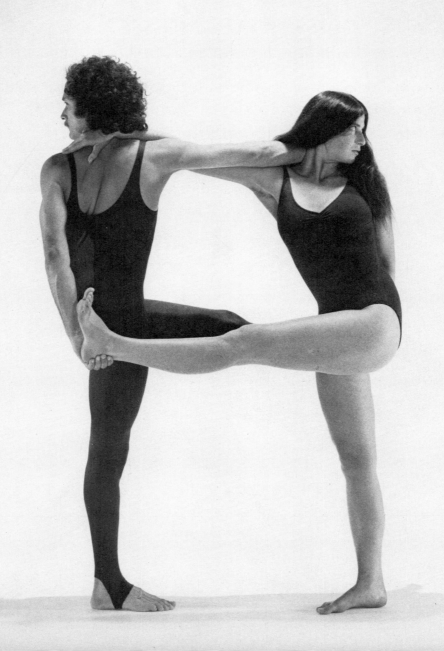

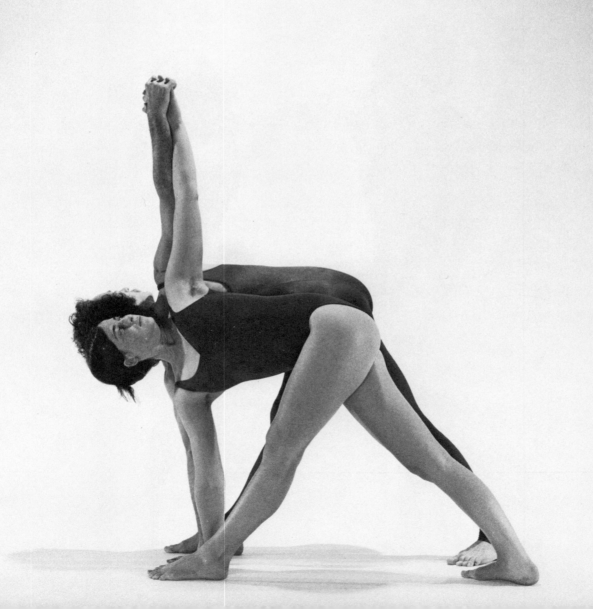

THE TWISTING TRIANGLE

Face your partner, standing ten inches apart, and spread your legs three feet. Turn your forward foot out straight and your back foot sixty degrees in, as shown. Make sure your front heel and toe are in line with your back foot arch. Extend your arms to shoulder level and hold your partner's hands. Both of you turn slowly toward the forward leg, bringing your rear arm between you to the front while your front arm moves over your head to the rear. This rotates the spine. Now, exhaling, extend the torso out and bring the palms or fingertips of your lower hand to the floor between the feet and turn your head to the ceiling. Keep the front feet even and adjust for differences in height with the rear feet. Use your hand clasp to get maximum extension vertically and press your shoulders together to get a good lengthening twist in the spine. The elbows of the upper arms can be interlocked to increase the stretch. Enjoy! Hold, then come out slowly in the same way you went into the pose, and smoothly turn to the other side.

BENEFITS: The twisting, extending action in this pose relieves tension and pressure on the spinal nerves. Done correctly, it feels wonderful. This pose stretches the leg muscles and opens the chest and shoulders. It increases the flow of nerve energy to the organs, improving digestion and elimination.

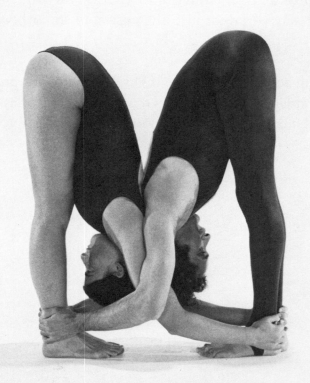

THE ANKLE LOCK I

Stand facing your partner about two feet apart. First one of you folds forward and then the other. Clasp each other's ankles, press your shoulders together, and then adjust the distance between the feet for a good stretch. To get the full effect of the pose, pull against your partner's ankles, bending your elbows and pressing your upper backs together to lengthen the spine. Do not hunch your shoulders or you will compress your neck. After holding, exhale and slowly lean your hips away from your partner's.

BENEFITS: This pose opens the shoulders and stretches the neck and leg muscles. Gripping your partner's ankles and pressing upper backs together allows you to stretch further and to hold the position more easily.

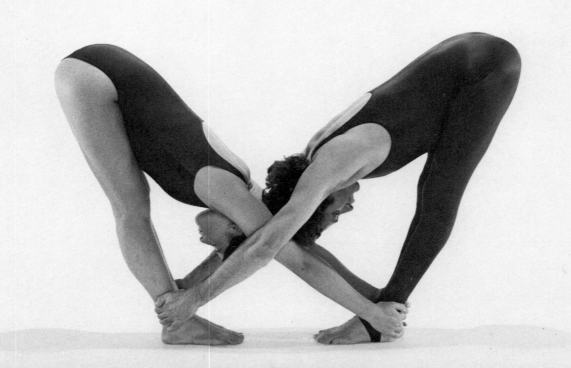

THE ANKLE LOCK II

Come into the Ankle Lock I pose. Hold your partner's ankles firmly and lean back to your maximum. Relax into the stretch so your spine extends from the tailbone to the neck. Keep your knees straight.

BENEFITS: By relaxing and letting gravity do the work in this variation, your spine gets a unique tension-relieving stretch. The shoulders are also worked and opened.

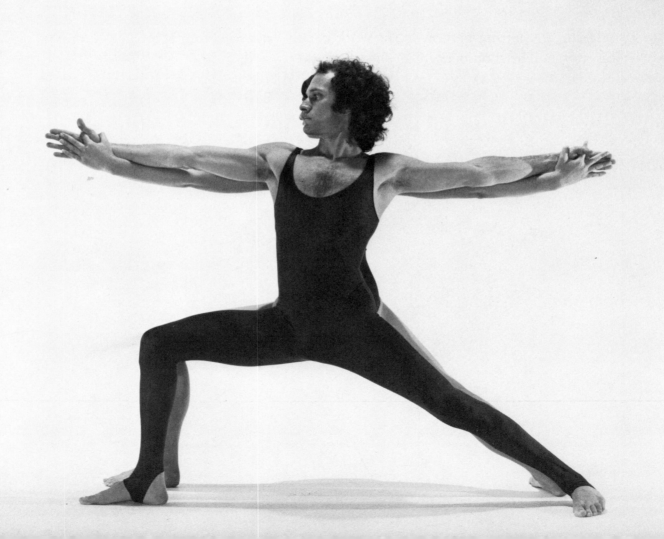

THE HERO I

Stand touching back to back with your legs spread four to five feet apart, holding hands and with arms extended to shoulder level. Turn the forward foot out and the rear foot in (see Photo 1). Keep the front feet even, exhale, and sink to a right angle, adjusting the distance between the feet with the rear leg. Take care not to lunge forward or rotate the hips. Tuck the tailbone down and press evenly against your partner's back and shoulders. Keep the chest open and lifted, the shoulders rolled back, and create another right angle between the thigh and torso (see Photo 6). Keep the outside of the rear foot pushing into the floor and the inner ankle lifted. Hold, breathing deeply, then straighten and smoothly change to the other side.

BENEFITS: This pose is a great strengthener and energizer, hence the name. It tones the nervous system, improves circulation and breathing, stretches the inner thighs, and firms the legs.

THE HERO II

Stand with the outer edges of the rear feet pressed together and your legs spread four to five feet apart. Clasp wrists while sinking to a right angle. Keep the wrists over the joined feet and maintain an even pull with the arms to add strength to the position and help overcome the tendency to lunge forward. Repeat on the other side.

BENEFITS: This pose helps correct a common error in the Hero I—failure to keep the torso erect and at a right angle to the thigh. The partners can use each other for leverage to increase the effects of the Hero II pose and get more lift in the chest.

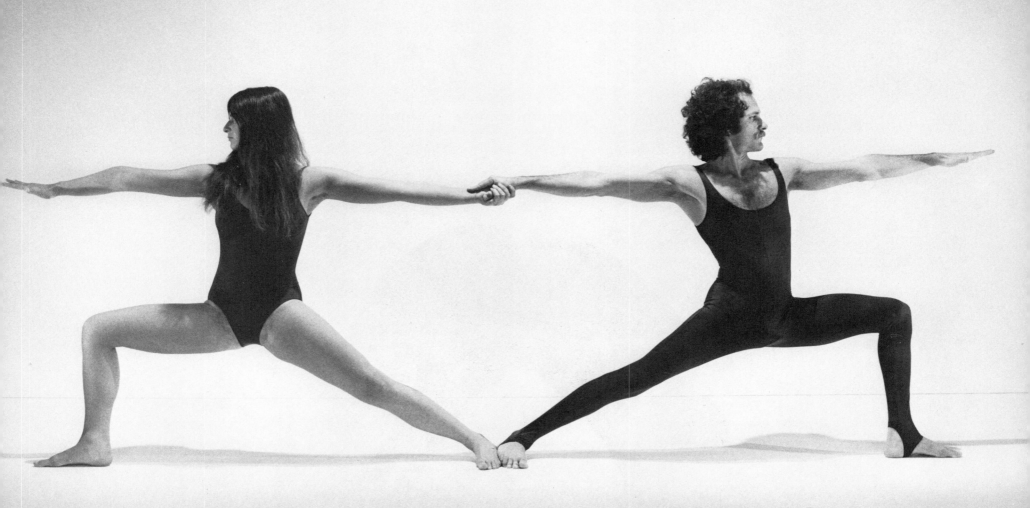

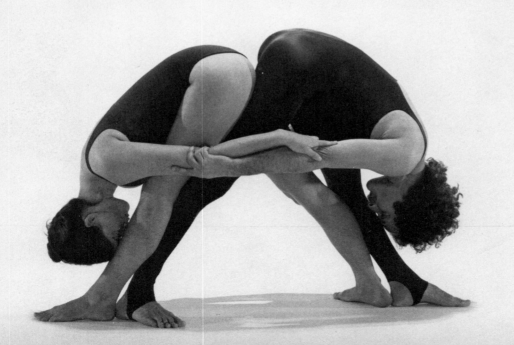

THE PYRAMID

Stand back to back in contact with your partner. One partner brings the left leg forward three feet as the other brings the right leg back three feet. Keep the outside edge of the rear foot pressed against your partner's heel. Reach back and hold each other's wrists. Then, exhaling, extend the trunk forward, sliding your hands up your partner's arms. Bend only as far as you can while keeping your back and legs straight. Press against your partner with feet firmly on the floor and pull with the arms to increase the extension of the spine and the stretch in the legs. Hold, come back up, then change sides by sliding the forward leg back and the back leg forward in unison with your partner.

BENEFITS: This pose gives a concentrated stretch to the back, buttock, and leg muscles, thus loosening the hip socket. The partners use the press of the legs and the pull of the arms to increase their ability to extend into the pose.

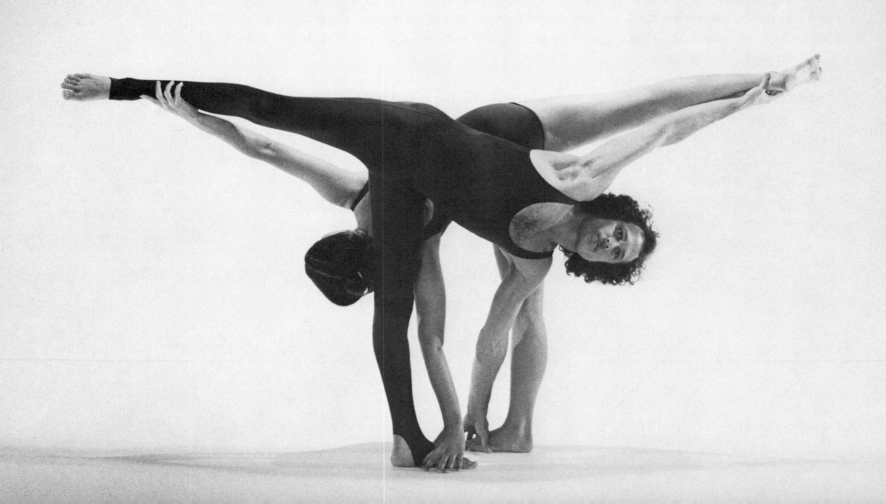

☀ THE FULL MOON

This pose is the double version of the classic Yoga Half Moon pose, therefore the name Full Moon. It is a little tricky in balance and foot position, so you may require some practice and experimentation before you can do it satisfactorily. Follow the instructions carefully. Stand back to back with your partner, ten inches apart. Both of you step three and one half feet to your right side with your right foot (which moves you in opposite directions because you are back to back). Then turn your left foot out and slide it back a few inches toward your right foot so your toes are in line with your partner's toes, yet your feet are still ten inches apart and parallel. Now come into the Triangle position (page 39), extending toward your partner over your left leg. Bend your left leg and extend your left hand over your partner's left foot, pressing the floor with your fingertips. Straighten your left leg as you raise your right until it is parallel with the floor. Grab the foot or calf of your partner's raised leg and roll your chest up and open. Look straight ahead or roll your head up to look at the ceiling. You must maintain steady attention on your balance and on your partner in order to hold this pose. Use your mutual support to roll hips and torso open to the maximum. Breathe smoothly, hold, then change sides.

BENEFITS: The Full Moon strengthens the legs and improves balance and concentration. It stretches open the pelvis and intercostal muscles. Because you have the support of a partner, you can extend and open more than you could if you did the Half Moon alone. This balancing pose will improve your attunement and sensitivity to your partner.

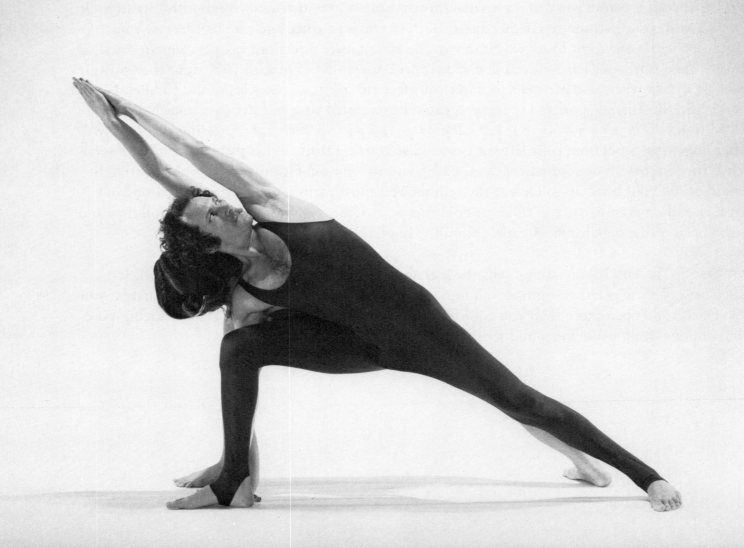

THE EXTENDED HERO

Come into the Hero I pose (page 61), keeping the forward feet about ten inches apart. Exhale and extend the trunk, dropping the leading arms between the feet (as shown), supporting yourself on your palm or fingertips. Extend the other arm over the head to touch your partner's palm. Keep the chest rolled open and facing as forward as possible. Notice the sides of the torso are kept parallel and the rear legs straight. When coming out of the pose, hold your partner's hands again and maintain the extension so that you come up straight and flow into the Hero pose. Hold the pose, breathing deeply, then straighten the legs, turn the opposite feet out, and repeat on the other side.

BENEFITS: The Extended Hero gives an excellent stretch to the top side of the body that should be felt from the fingertips to the heels. It tones the legs and increases strength.

THE HERO BALANCE

Stand about four feet apart facing each other. Exhaling, stretch forward. Hold hands and bring the torso parallel to the floor, sliding your hands up to your partner's shoulders and raising your back leg so that it is parallel to the floor. Keep your hips level, facing the floor. In the photo both partners are balanced on the same leg (left is shown), which adds stability to the pose. See if you can extend forward far enough to bring a *slight* curve to the spine. Look at the floor or into each other's eyes. Hold, breathing evenly, then change sides.

BENEFITS: This pose strengthens the lumbar region, stomach, inner legs, and ankles. It teaches you to stand on the whole foot and improves balance. Bracing against a partner aids you in stretching into the pose.

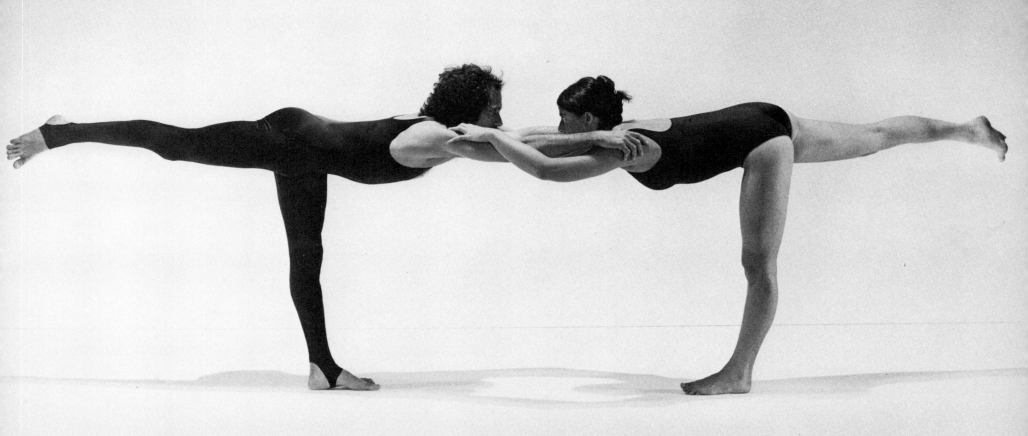

THE SPLIT MUSHROOM

Bend forward from the Pump pose (page 49), exhaling, and slide your hands up your partner's arms as far as you can. Keep your spine extending, legs straight, and feet pressing evenly on the floor. Hold until the leg and back muscles are stretched.

BENEFITS: Bending forward with the head down increases circulation and the flow of oxygen to the brain. This pose banishes fatigue and lengthens the same muscles as the Pump pose.

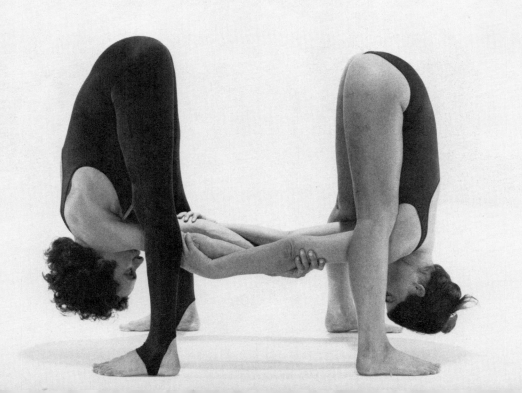

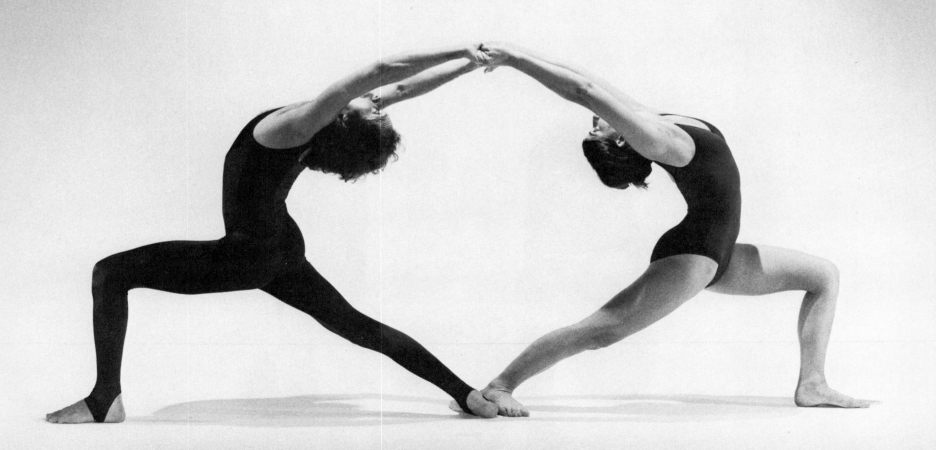

✸ THE DIAMOND HERO

Using the same leg as your partner (right to right or left to left), stand with feet pointing in opposite directions, outside edges touching. Spread your legs four to five feet apart, turning your forward foot perpendicular to your rear foot. Extend your arms out to the side and reach back to hold your partner's hands. Keep your hips facing forward and slowly sink to a right angle, exhaling as you raise your arms over your head, arch your back and neck. You may have to experiment and adjust the distance between your feet in order to achieve the right-angle position. Press against your partner's foot firmly to create more lift along the spine. Keep your chest lifted and tailbone tucked down so you feel the stretch and movement of energy from your foot all the way to your head. Repeat on the other side.

BENEFITS: The Diamond Hero is a highly invigorating pose because it creates a flow of nerve energy in the spine. This pose helps correct rounding of the upper back and improves the mobility of the shoulder joints.

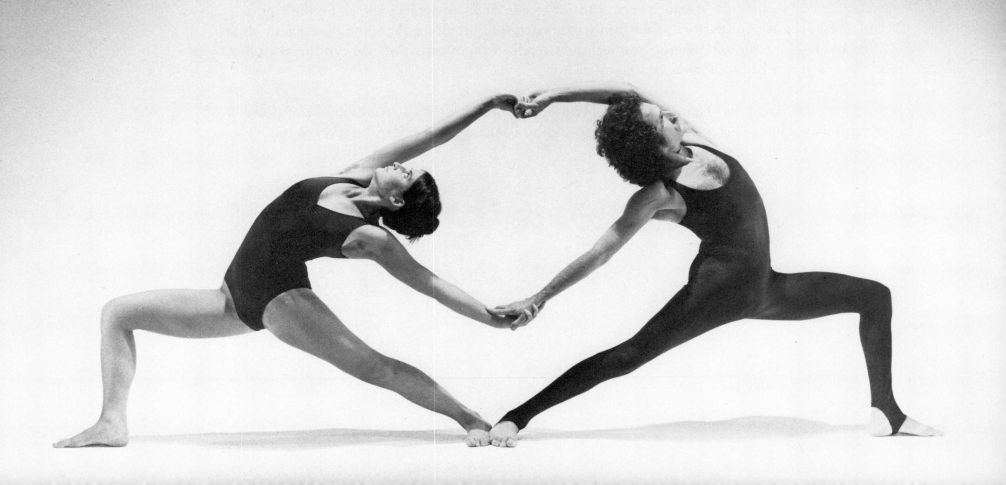

THE TWISTING DIAMOND HERO

Come into the Hero II (page 62). Bend sideways, exhaling, and bring your upper arm over your head to grab your partner's hand. Twist so that your arms, legs, and shoulders are on the same plane and lift your upper ribs toward the ceiling. Press your feet together and feel the stretch along the leg and up the torso. Hold a short time, come back to the Hero II, straighten, and then change sides. If you are unable to do the pose in this way, try it without the right angle by keeping your forward leg straight.

BENEFITS: This pose gives lateral flexibility to the spine. It also strengthens and opens the intercostal muscles and stretches the pelvic area and tones the abdominal muscles and organs.

❋ THE TWISTING HERO

Stand twelve inches apart facing each other with your legs spread four to five feet and the arms extended out at shoulder level. Holding hands, rotate as explained in the Twisting Triangle pose (page 55). Then sink to a right angle. Bring the lower arm over the knee and place the hand on the floor to the outside of the foot. Press shoulders with your partner and use the upper arms to lift and twist to the maximum. Your upper elbows may be interlocked to increase the stretch. Keep your rear leg straight and don't collapse the chest. Hold the pose, breathing evenly, then straighten and change to the other side.

BENEFITS: The twist and extension relieves compression and pain in the lumbar region. It improves digestion and relieves gastric problems.

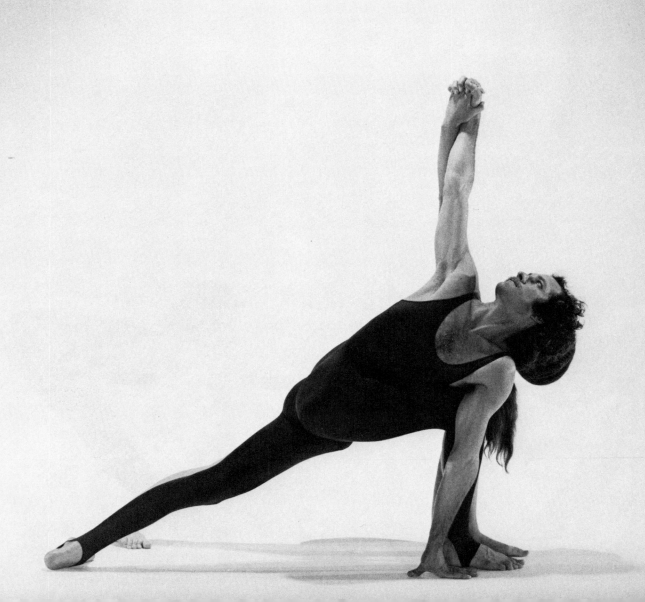

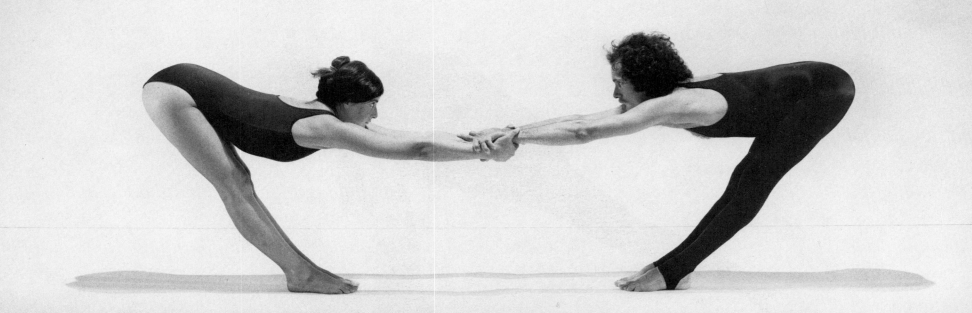

THE SUSPENSION BRIDGE

Face your partner at a distance of four feet. With your feet together and legs straight, bend from the hips and clasp your partner's hands. Exhale and lean into the stretch, letting your hips move back while your spine extends forward.

BENEFITS: The Suspension Bridge is excellent for relieving pressure along the spine because it creates space between the vertebrae. It stretches and removes stiffness and tension from the muscles of the back, the backs of the legs, and the shoulders. It feels great too!

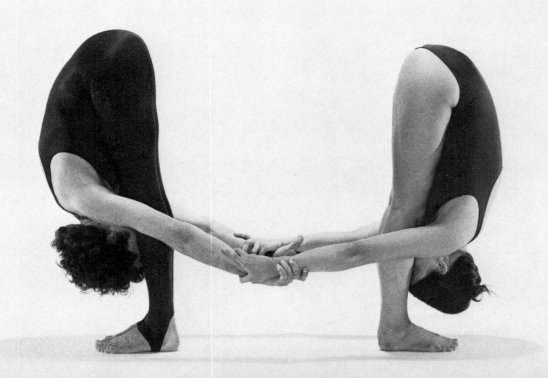

THE LINKED FORWARD FOLD

Stand back to back about three feet apart. Fold forward, exhaling, and reach back to clasp your partner's wrists. You may have to adjust your distance, depending on your flexibility. Stretch into this position and slowly move your head toward your feet, elongating the spine. Keep elbows and knees straight. As a variation for more flexible students, after holding this pose, inhale, then exhale slowly as you lean apart and deeper into the stretch. Stay attentive to each other, holding wrists firmly and keeping the pull even.

BENEFITS: Holding hands allows both partners to increase their forward stretch. The Linked Forward Fold overcomes the negative effects of sitting and helps prevent leg cramps. It increases the stretch of the leg muscles and lengthens the Achilles tendon. The pose also removes residual tension, uneven pulling on the skeleton, relieves sciatica and lower-back pain, and improves digestion.

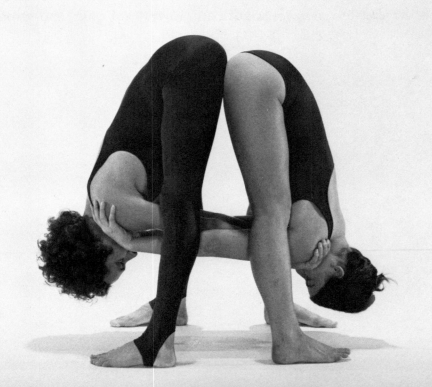

☀ THE MUSHROOM I

After holding the Split Mushroom (page 72), move closer together until your buttocks meet. You each slide your hands up your partner's arms, all the way to the shoulders if possible, and pull the other gently forward.

BENEFITS: By leaning on and holding one another, you are able to relax and stretch the muscles further.

☀ THE MUSHROOM II

Stand back to back with your feet together, about one foot from your partner. As you exhale, bend forward, pressing the buttocks together, and grab your ankles. Extend your spine down and forward, but keep your head arched back. Then reach back to grab your partner's shoulders. (To do this, you may have to adjust the distance between your feet.) Use the pull on the shoulders and the pressing at the buttocks to stretch into the position. Keep your neck elongated.

BENEFITS: This pose is both aesthetic and enjoyable. It gives you all the benefits of forward bending and greatly increases the extension of the lower back and the length of the hamstrings as you press against your partner.

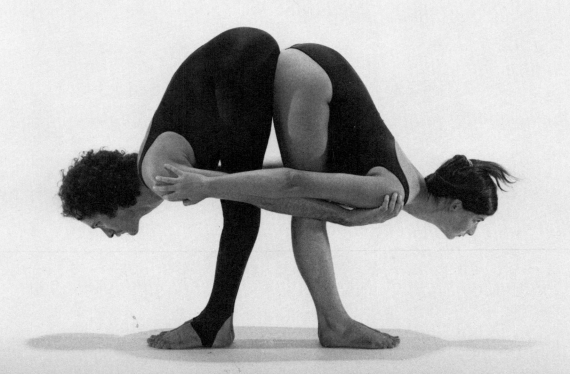

☀ THE STANDING TORTOISE

First one partner comes into position by standing with the legs spread about two feet apart, bending forward until the shoulders are between the legs, and placing the hands on the floor behind the feet. Then the other partner assumes the pose and moves in closer until both partners' backs gently touch. Each then bends the knees slightly and reaches through the legs and around to hold hands as shown. Hold tightly and straighten the knees as much as possible.

BENEFITS: The Standing Tortoise is an advanced pose that gives an intense stretch to the inner thighs and sharpens your sense of balance.

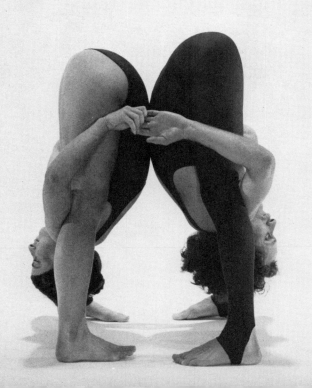

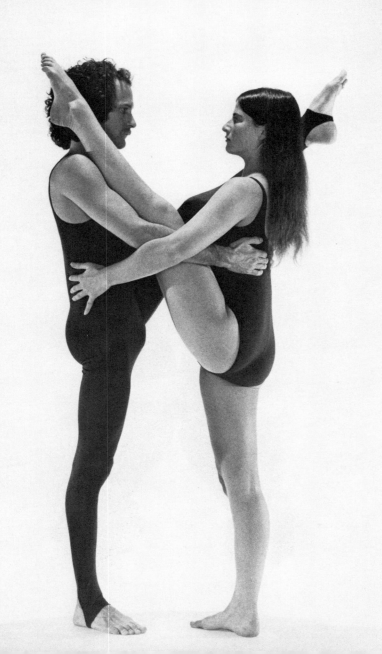

☀ THE SCISSORS

Stand one to two feet apart. Assist one another in raising the left leg onto the other's right shoulder. Hold each other at the waist for support and lift your torso. Keep your knees as straight as possible and pull closer together for increased stretch. Hold, then change sides. If you are unable to get your leg onto your partner's shoulder, stand farther apart and hold hands instead of waists.

BENEFITS: The Scissors stretches the legs and strengthens the ankles. It improves balance and prepares you for the full splits.

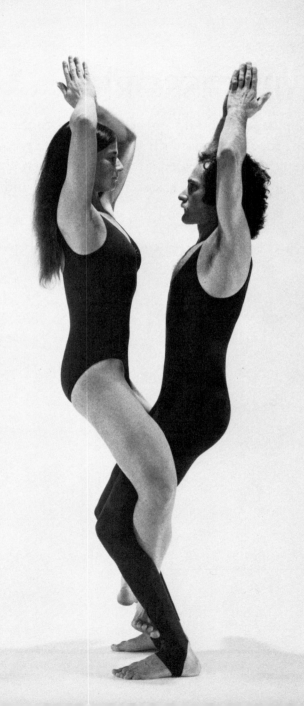

☀ SHIVA-SHAKTI

This position has been used by dancers in India to depict the play of matter—the cosmic male principle (Shiva)—and energy—the cosmic female principle (Shakti). Shiva stands with legs spread two feet apart, bending about forty-five degrees at the knees. Shakti wraps one leg around Shiva's thigh and hooks her toes around his shinbone. Then, supporting herself by holding his shoulders, Shakti wraps her other leg around Shiva's thigh. Both partners then raise their palms over the head in salute. After holding, you may change roles if your partner is strong enough to bear your weight.

BENEFITS: This position greatly strengthens the back, legs, and knees.

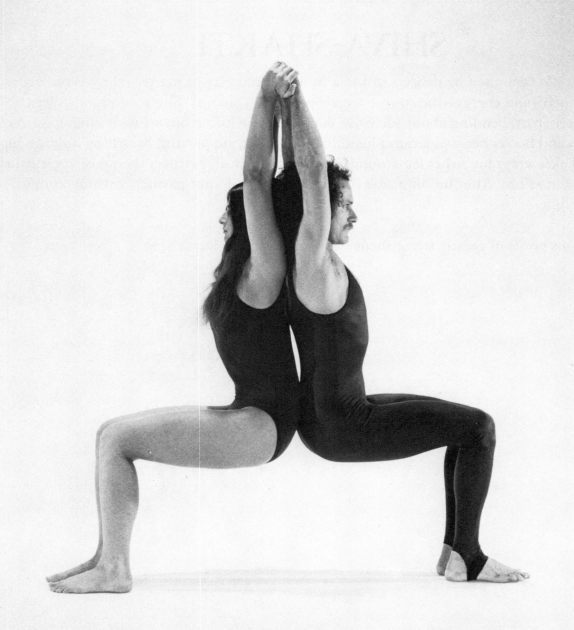

THE CHAIR

Stand with your back pressing as evenly as possible against your partner's and clasp your hands overhead as shown. Slowly sink, being careful to maintain even pressure, while walking the feet forward until the legs are bent at right angles. Keep your legs together, your backs straight and evenly pressed together with the tailbones tucked down. Before you try this with your partner, practice with your back against a wall.

BENEFITS: The Chair improves posture, straightens the shoulders, and strengthens the knees and thighs. This pose teaches you how to keep balanced with your partner, and so develops sensitivity and attuned concentration—a good lesson for any close relationship.

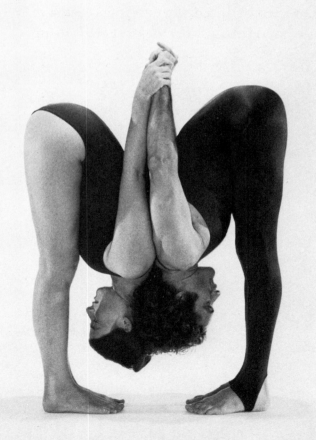

THE FACING FORWARD FOLD

One at a time bend forward from the hips and place your hands on the floor for support. Move closer until you can press your upper backs together as you extend your heads down toward the floor. Then raise your arms behind your backs, clasp hands, and lift, pulling the shoulders open.

BENEFITS: By locking the partners into position, this pose allows you to maintain an increased stretch. The Facing Forward Fold corrects any tendency to rounded shoulders and lengthens the hamstrings.

Assisting Poses

THE HIP-SUPPORTED BACK STRETCH I

Stand back to back and hook elbows firmly. Have your partner bend forward slowly, sensitive to the movement of your spine. Relax as you are bent over. When you are lowered back down, continue into a forward bend and ease your partner into a back bend. The point of emphasis may be changed by sliding the hip support higher or lower on the spine.

BENEFITS: This pose puts a natural traction on the spine. As you exhale and relax into the stretch, tensions and pressures are released. The Hip-Supported Back Stretch I makes the back supple.

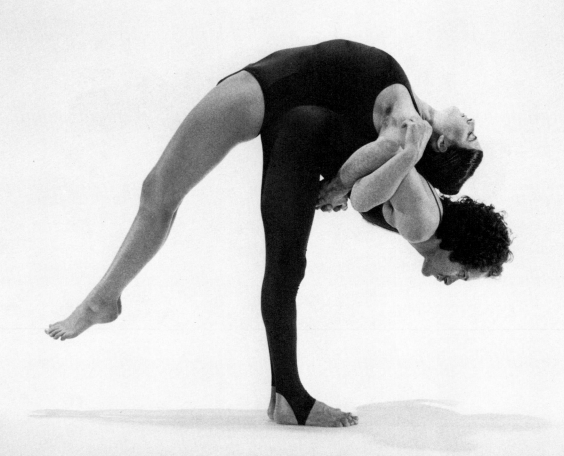

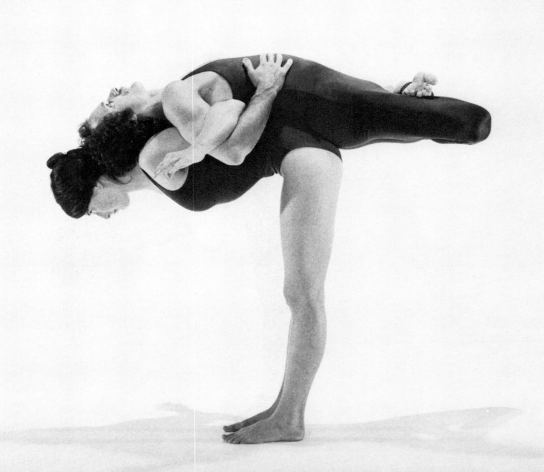

THE HIP-SUPPORTED BACK STRETCH II

To do this pose, you must be able to bring your legs into the Lotus without using your hands. Follow the instructions for the Hip-Supported Back Stretch I and fold your legs into the Lotus after you are stretched over backward. You will experience a different kind of stretch.

BENEFITS: This pose combines the benefits of the Lotus with those of the Hip-Supported Back Stretch I. The muscles in the front of the pelvis and top of the thighs get increased stretch.

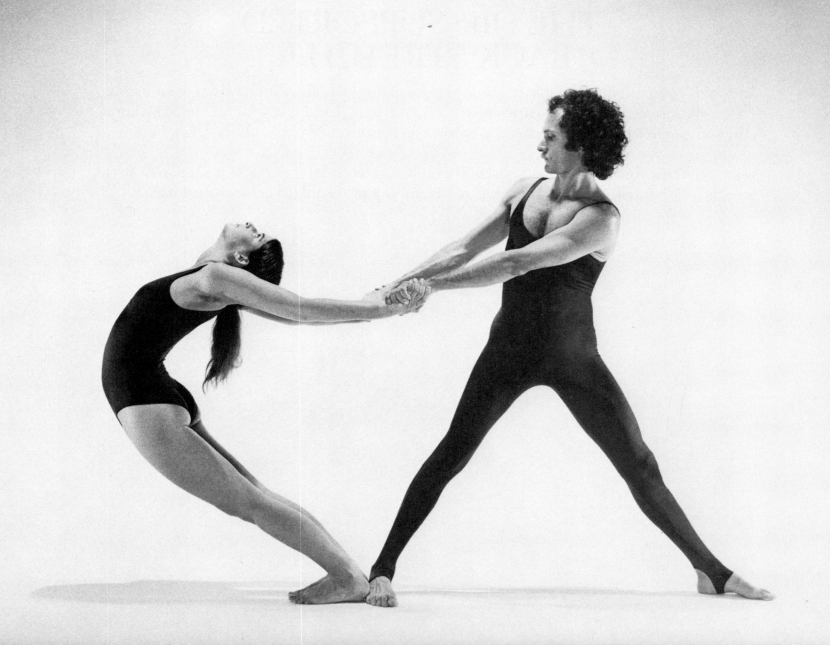

THE ARM-SUPPORTED BACK BEND

One partner stands straight, feet together, with heels braced against the outer edge of the other partner's foot, as shown. Reach back to clasp wrists. Then arch forward, pressing the feet firmly on the ground. Lean into the stretch while extending the muscles along the backs of the legs, tucking the tailbone down, and raising the chest to make the spine long. Follow this pose with the Arm-Supported Forward Fold.

BENEFITS: This pose expands the chest, back, and shoulders. Being supported and suspended allows you to use gravity to get more stretch. The Arm-Supported Back Bend warms up the back muscles and strengthens the lumbar region and hips.

THE ARM-SUPPORTED
FORWARD FOLD

Assume the Arm-Supported Back Bend pose. Continue holding your partner's wrists and bend forward, keeping your back flat and extended while moving into a complete forward fold. Lean firmly on your partner's arms to gain the full benefit of this pose.

BENEFITS: As you hang from your partner's arms your calves get a good stretch and your lumbar region and neck are relaxed and lengthened, which releases tension. This pose helps to develop trust in your partner.

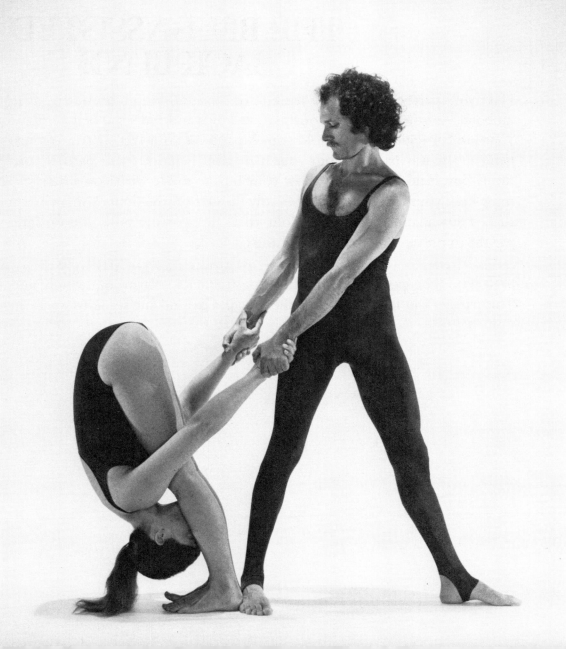

THE BELT-ASSISTED
BACK BEND

Have your partner take a long flat belt or rope and loop it around your hips just above the tailbone. As you bend back your partner holds and pulls the belt firmly to take any strain off your lumbar region and to hold your hips above your feet. If you are flexible enough, you may bend all the way back and put your hands on the floor. Your partner continues to hold the belt firmly but, if necessary, may allow your hips to move with you a little as you bend back. You must keep your feet parallel and evenly pressed on the floor, knees close together, tailbone tucked down, and chest lifted. Hold, then your partner pulls you up carefully, supporting your weight to prevent any straining of the back.

BENEFITS: This pose allows the bending partner to warm up, stretch, and strengthen the back. This partner can lean back onto the belt and extend the spine to open the chest and shoulders.

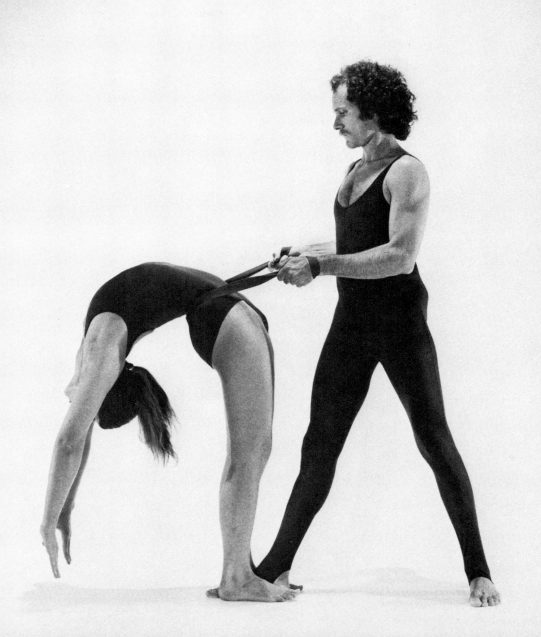

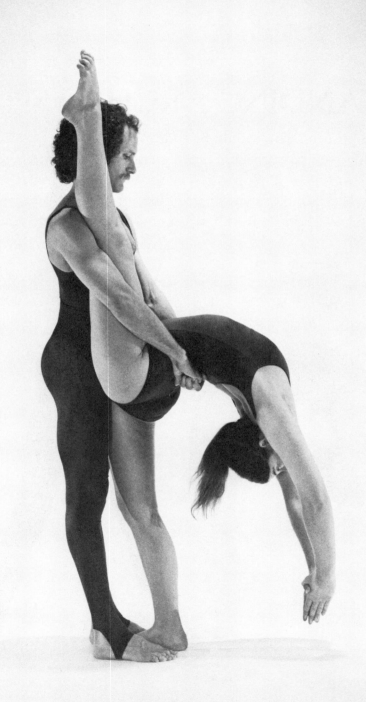

✸ THE STANDING ARCHED SPLIT

Before attempting to do this position, you should be thoroughly warmed up and able to do the Splits (page 182) easily. Facing your partner, raise one leg onto the shoulder. Have your partner clasp hands around your lumbar region for support. Then move in close, bracing your thighs firmly against your partner's. Holding on to your partner's arms, lift your chest and bend back. Then let go and slowly extend your arms out only when you feel strong and ready. Repeat on the other side.

BENEFITS: The Standing Arched Split gives an intense stretch to the legs that fully lengthens the muscles, while allowing the back to be stretched with protective support. The chest, arms, and shoulders are strongly opened.

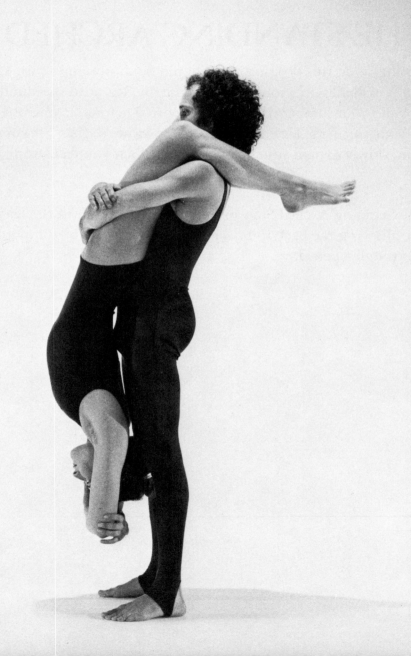

☀ THE HANGING YOGI

Face your partner and place both palms on the floor, shoulder distance apart. Keep the arms straight and swing the legs up in the air while your partner stands to the side behind you and catches your legs (careful!). Then bend your knees over your partner's shoulders. Have your partner clasp arms over your legs. When you feel firmly supported, fold your arms above your head. Relax, breathe deeply, and hang, letting gravity stretch the vertebrae. *Note:* If you cannot get up this way, then do the Head Stand (page 137), bend your knees over your partner's shoulders, and push up with your hands as your partner lifts you.

BENEFITS: This pose feels wonderful. It provides a soothing stretch and natural traction for the spine. Hang out and enjoy!

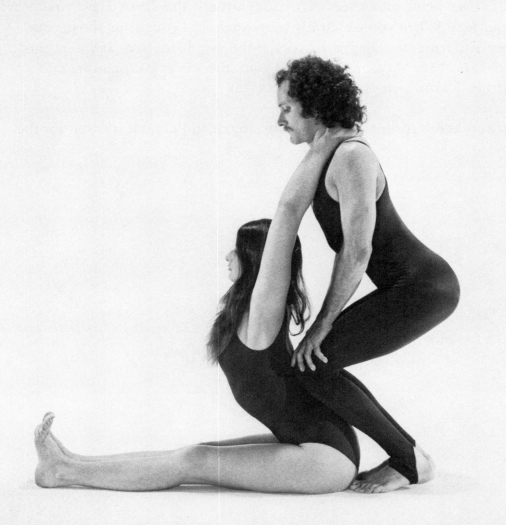

THE BACK STRETCHER I

Sit with your legs together and extended in front as your partner stands close behind you and places bent knees into your back, as shown. Reach up and clasp your hands around your partner's neck. Your partner then braces with arms on knees and stretches you up. Allow your spine to be pushed forward as you are lifted. Your buttocks should remain on the floor and your feet flexed for a deep stretch.

BENEFITS: The hamstrings and pelvic muscles are lengthened and the shoulders and upper spine are opened and stretched forward in this pose. It prepares you to move correctly in forward bends.

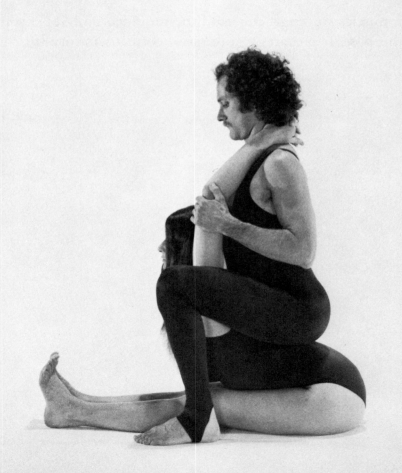

THE BACK STRETCHER II

One partner comes into the Forward Fold pose (page 167). The other sits lightly on the center of the floor partner's back, bending forward so the other can reach up and clasp hands around the neck. Now stretch your partner into the pose, increasing the weight on the back by sitting down as you straighten your torso.

BENEFITS: This pose gives a stronger stretch than the Back Stretcher I. It creates an intense opening in the chest, shoulders, triceps, and intercostal muscles and also fully stretches the legs and lower back. Short hamstrings often limit flexibility in forward bending, and this is a very good pose for lengthening them.

THE FORWARD PULL

Sit in the Forward Fold (page 167) with your partner standing in front of you and press your feet against your partner's shinbones. Clasp wrists, keeping your legs together and straight. Then the standing partner arches and leans back to pull and stretch you forward. Hold, then change positions with your partner.

BENEFITS: In forward bending it is difficult to achieve the correct extension of the lower back and pelvis. This pose pulls your tight back muscles and hamstrings to assist you in accomplishing the correct movement. At the same time your partner is able to get a supported stretch in a back bend.

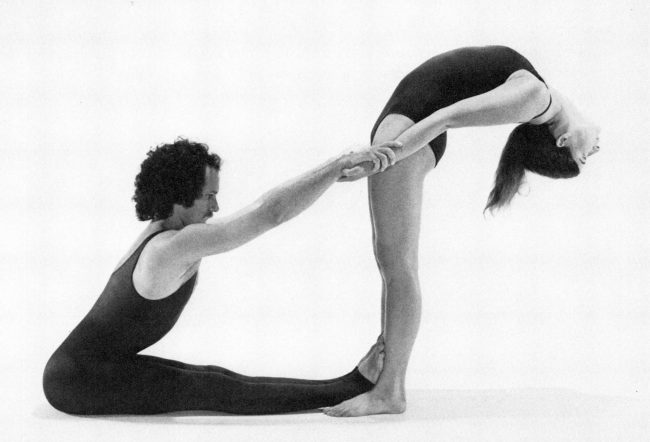

THE HORSE

This pose is not as difficult as it looks and can be done by most beginners, as long as your partner is not too heavy for you. Bend forward at the hips and hold on to a waist-level table, ledge, or chair. Your partner then carefully sits on your back close to your hips. Keep your legs straight and back relaxed, allowing your partner's weight to stretch your muscles. As you become more flexible, the stretch can be increased by having your partner slowly slide farther up your back, balancing by extending the arms overhead and hooking the ankles, as shown.

BENEFITS: The Horse gives a wonderful stretch to the spine, shoulders, triceps, and legs, with emphasis on the thoracic vertebrae and hamstrings. The weight of your partner elongates your muscles, tendons, and ligaments to relieve tension and increase mobility.

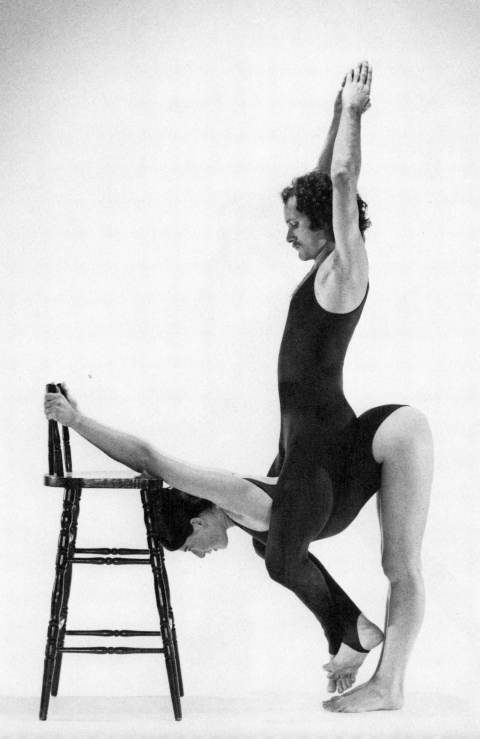

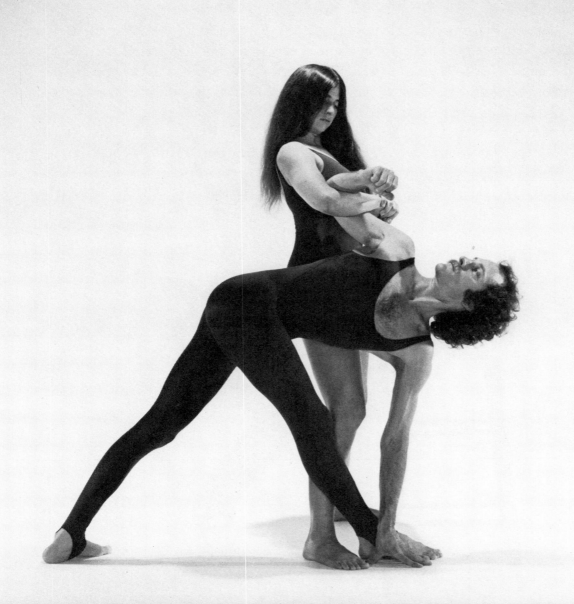

THE TWIST ASSIST

One partner comes into the Twisting Triangle pose (page 55). The assisting partner then steps in behind and you interlock right elbows, as shown, while the assisting partner presses the hip into the twisting partner's middle back. Then the assisting partner slowly begins pulling the other's elbow and increasing the pressure of the hip in the back to rotate the chest into an open position and extend the spine. Repeat on the other side.

BENEFITS: This assisting pose adjusts the vertebrae and alleviates pressure on the nerves. It releases compression in the lower back and allows you to get more rotation.

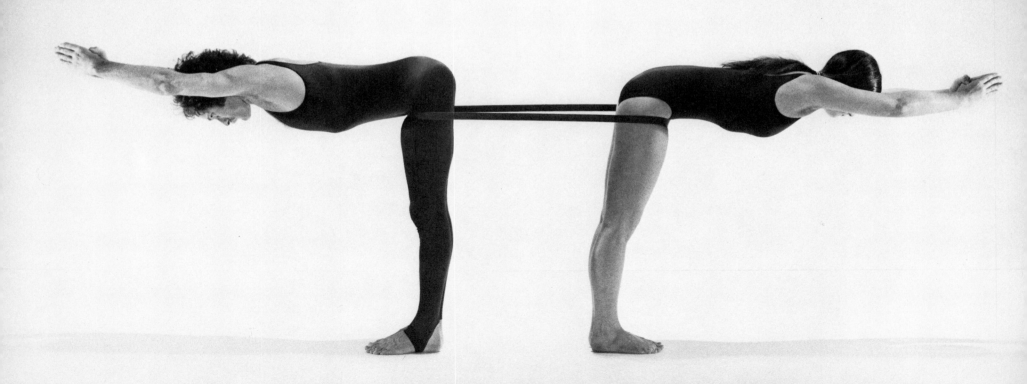

Back Bend Poses

THE ROPE EXTENSION STRETCH

This position is done by slowly and steadily increasing pressure on the belt, so keen attention is necessary. Use a four- to five-foot strong belt or rope loop. Both partners stand inside it far enough apart to make it taut. Keep your feet together and adjust the belt so that it is on the top of the thigh, under the pelvic bone. Extend the arms up over the head with palms together and begin to bend forward, keeping the pressure on the belt even. Continue to bend until your torso is parallel to the floor, using the pull of the belt to get increased extension. Use this position to warm up the muscles before doing back bends.

BENEFITS: The Rope Extension Stretch is excellent for strengthening the back. Partners must maintain equal pressure on the belt, which develops attuned concentration.

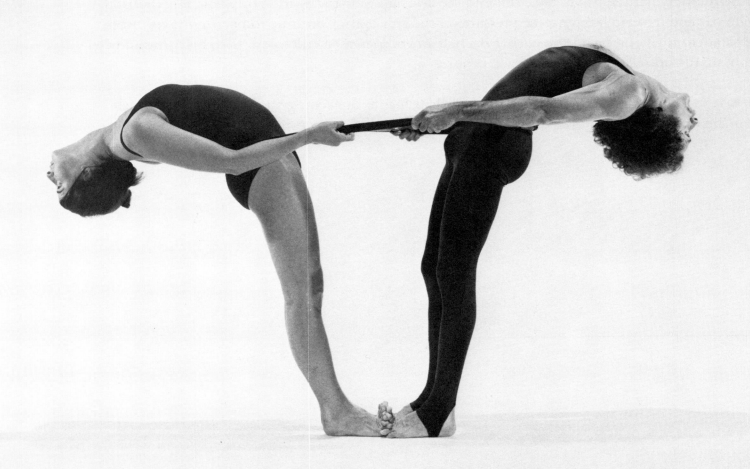

THE BELT-LINKED BACK BEND

This pose requires even more balanced pressure and sensitive attunement to your partner than the Rope Extension Stretch, which should be learned first. Stand with feet together, toes bent back and pressing, as shown. Grab the belt and begin bending back slightly, maintaining equal pressure. Then hold until the pose becomes steady. Now continue to bend backward as you lift your sternum. Keeping the pressure perfectly even on the belt, press the floor harder with your feet until you feel the lift along your legs up to your chest. The tailbone should be tucked down and the legs kept straight.

BENEFITS: This pose strengthens and opens the back and intercostal muscles. It also improves balance, attunement, and concentration.

THE FOUNTAIN

Stand with your feet together and your toes pressing against each other's, as shown. Clasp wrists and lean back, straightening the elbows and tucking the tailbone down. Maintain an even pull with the arms and bend back carefully so that you can feel a lifting of the chest and a movement of energy from your feet to your head. Hold, breathe evenly, and repeat two times.

BENEFITS: The Fountain emphasizes lifting and opening the upper back, chest, and sternum. It strengthens the back and buttock muscles and helps overcome rounding in the shoulders.

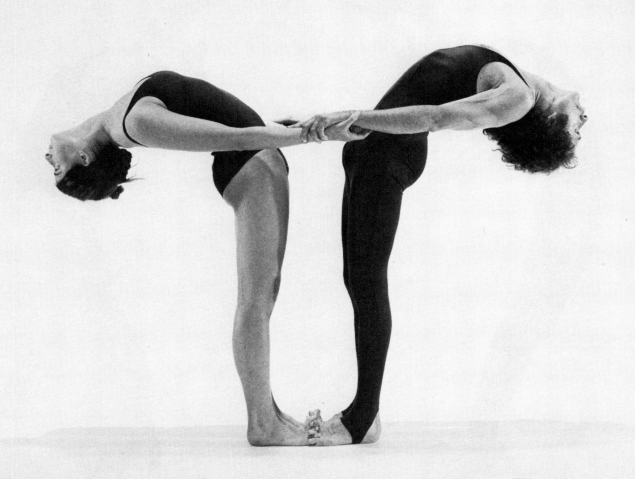

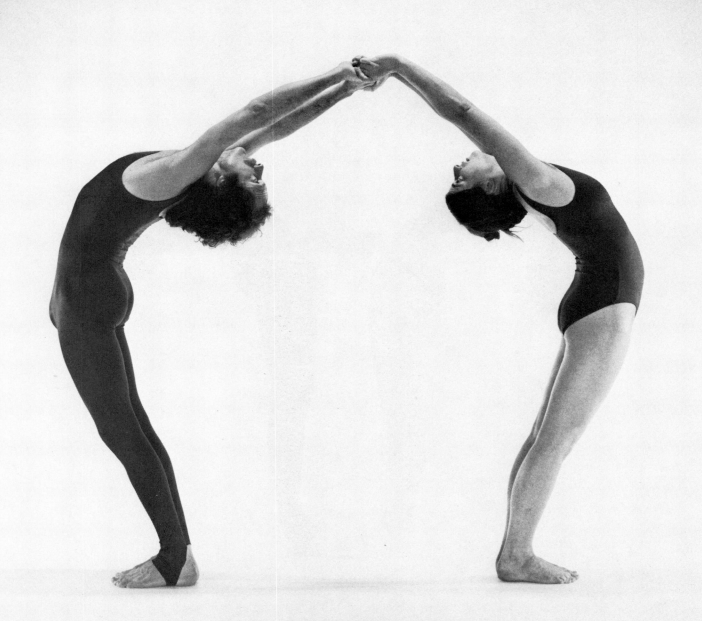

THE ARCHWAY

Stand back to back about three feet from each other with your feet together. Bring your arms overhead to clasp hands. Then straighten your arms and begin arching back, tucking the tailbone down and leaning out into the stretch. Use your arms to pull yourself up and keep your knees straight. Breathe evenly. Hold a few moments, rest, then repeat.

BENEFITS: The lift of the arms assists in getting an extension in the spine. This pose warms up, strengthens, stretches, and tones the back muscles.

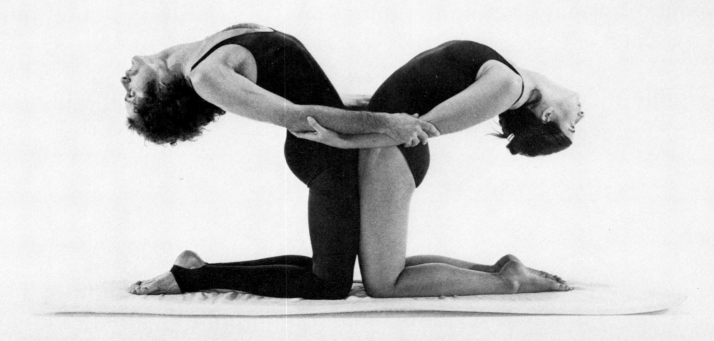

THE CAMEL

Kneel on a mat or carpet with your knees together and press your thighs against your partner's thighs. Clasp your partner's arms and arch back, pressing your hips together while lifting the chest. Use the pull on your arms to get maximum lifting and stretching movement. Hold, breathing evenly, then repeat. Rest by sitting back on your heels and placing your forehead on the mat.

BENEFITS: The Camel brings flexibility to the spine. It opens the intercostal muscles, increases breathing capacity, and stretches the back, thighs, and pelvis. By pressing each other at the hips and thighs the muscles of the lower back are protected from injury.

THE CRESCENT MOON I

Stand back to back about four feet apart. Bend the right knee and bring the left leg back under your partner's thigh with the heel raised until the ball of your foot presses your partner's heel. Arch back and reach up to clasp hands. Sink your hips down and forward as you use your arms to stretch the torso up. Keep your forward foot flat and pressing firmly down. Hold, breathing evenly, then change legs.

BENEFITS: The Crescent Moon I stretches the tops of the thighs and pelvis, lengthens the Achilles tendons, and opens the upper back and shoulders. It energizes the nervous system and increases mobility of the back.

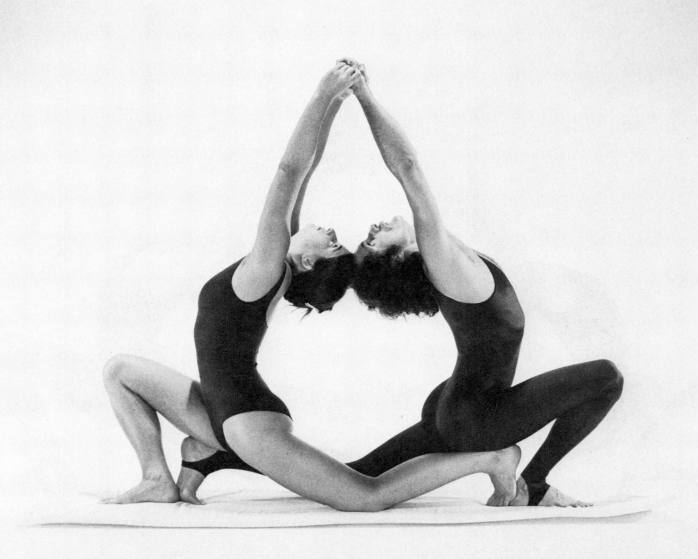

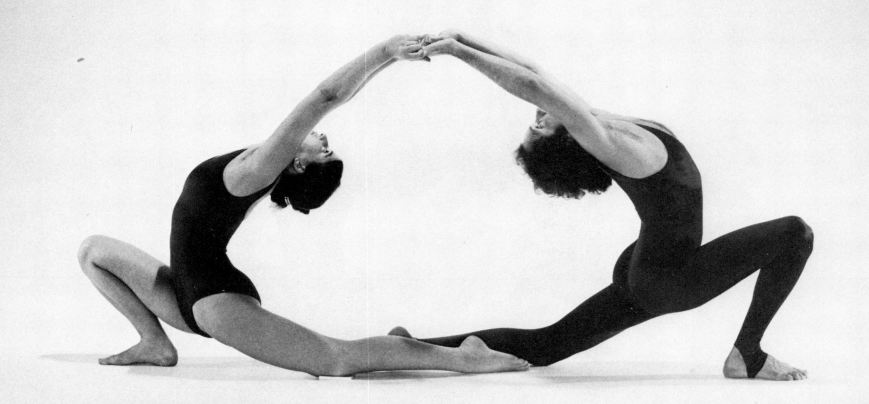

☀ THE CRESCENT MOON II

After holding Crescent Moon I, release your hand grip, point the rear foot, and slide a little farther away from your partner. The farther apart you slide the more intense the stretch will become. Sink your hips as much as possible and arch back to clasp each other's wrists. Hold, then change legs.

BENEFITS: This pose stretches the thighs, pelvis, and back muscles. It lengthens the Achilles tendons, opens the shoulders, and is invigorating.

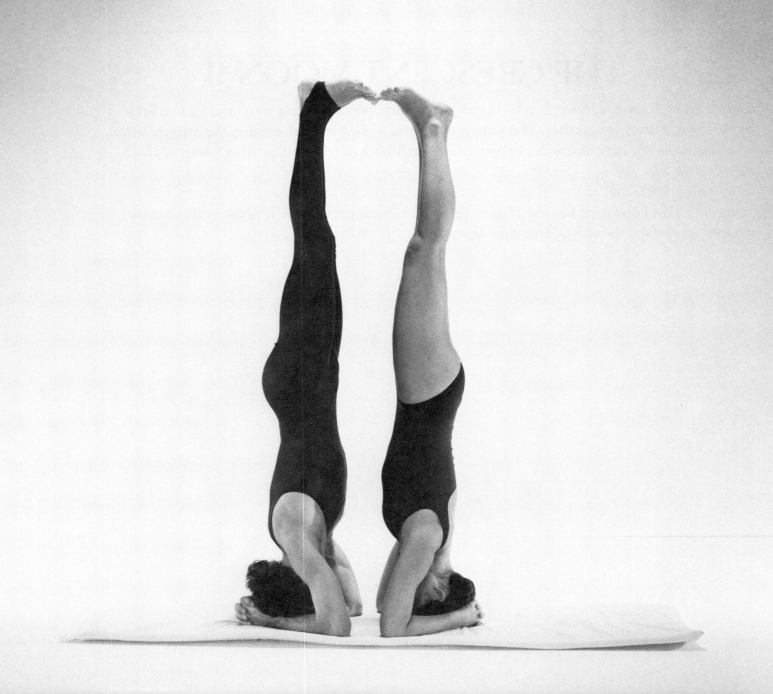

Inverted Poses

☀ THE HEAD STAND

Both partners should be proficient at the Head Stand alone before trying it together. If a competent teacher is not available, practice near a wall or with your partner's assistance. In the Head Stand most of the body's weight is supported along the forearms. The elbows are kept one forearm's width apart and the top of the head is placed on the mat. Keep your shoulders lifted *away* from your ears to make your neck longer, thereby keeping pressure off the vertebrae. Come into the double Head Stand one at a time. After the first partner is steady, the second comes into position by placing the head and arms on the mat and the legs out to each side of the partner. Then slowly raise the legs up. Practice this farther apart at first, then move closer together. Slowly increase your time up to ten minutes in this pose to get more benefit. Breathe evenly. When you are both very steady in this pose, you may begin to learn leg movements. Bring your legs in contact with your partner's legs and slowly move and stretch in a scissorslike motion, the right leg moving forward while the left moves back. Alternate legs a few times, then take turns gently spreading each other's legs out to the sides by pressing your feet on your partner's toes or ankles.

BENEFITS: The Head Stand is the king of Yoga poses and a fountain of youth. Gravity is a major factor in the aging process. By reversing the pull of gravity on the body, sluggish blood is drained back to the heart and lungs. The brain receives an increased flow of blood, oxygen, and *prana,* which improves concentration and mental clarity. The pineal and pituitary glands, internal organs, and diaphragm are toned. The face, scalp, and eyes receive increased circulation. The arms, shoulders, back muscles, and legs are strengthened. The Head Stand makes one feel young, strong, and vital. In the double Head Stand you are able to use your partner for reference and concentration and it is easier to hold the pose longer.

✺ THE FOLDED LOTUS
HEAD STAND

Come into the Head Stand and place your legs in the Half Lotus or Lotus. Now one at a time fold your Lotus down to your chest. Or, if possible, touch your knees and fold down together. Then press evenly against your partner, being careful not to knock each other over. Keep the shoulders lifted and the spine extended. Hold a few moments, raise up, maintaining the Lotus position, and then repeat.

BENEFITS: This pose improves balance and concentration in the Head Stand. By pressing together, you are able to increase the flexibility and strength of the lower back.

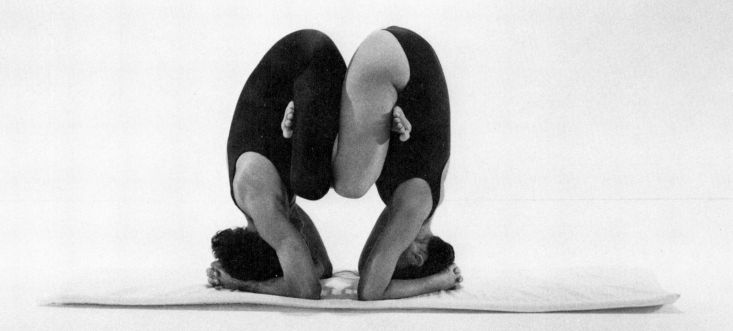

☀ THE ARROWHEAD SCORPION

Kneel facing your partner and place your forearms parallel at shoulder width, touching your partner's fingertips. Bend the head back *without cramping the neck* and carefully raise the legs one at a time. Push down with the forearms, lift the shoulders, and extend upward. When you are balanced, bring your feet together, pressing steadily so as not to knock your friend over. (Partners of different sizes may bring feet to calf.) After holding, come down and rest in the kneeling position.

BENEFITS: The Arrowhead Scorpion develops and tones the arms, shoulders, back, and stomach. It creates a surge of energy and leaves you feeling strong and vigorous.

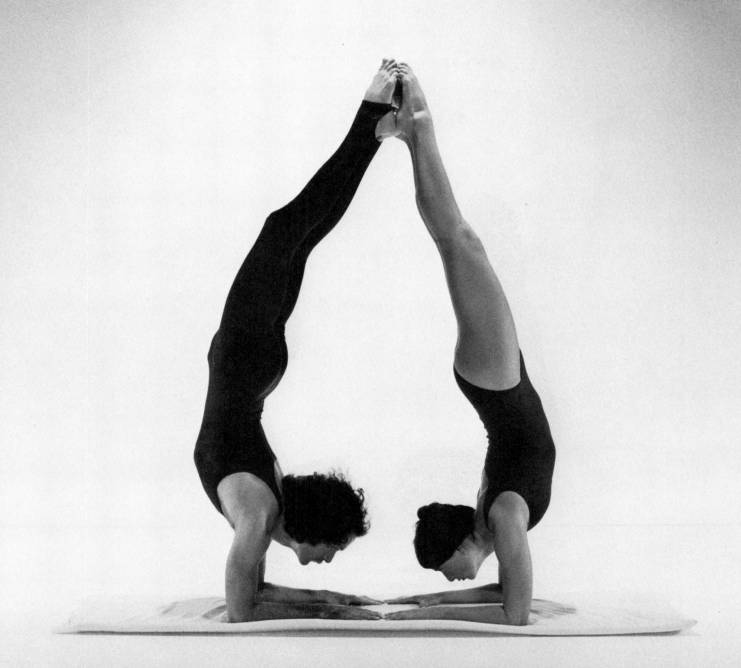

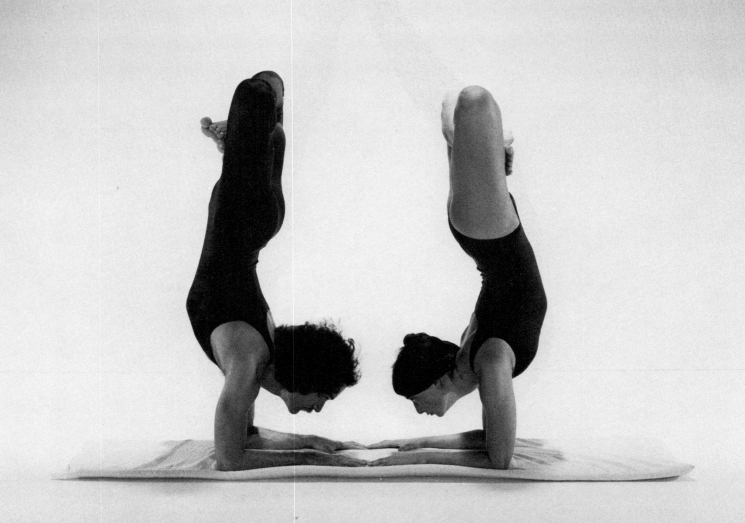

☀ THE LOTUS SCORPION I

To do this pose, you must be able to balance steadily and bring your legs into the Lotus without using your arms. After raising up into the Scorpion, come into the Lotus position.

BENEFITS: While this pose provides no mutual physical support, it gives mental support and is aesthetic, enjoyable, and increases stamina and concentration. It prepares you for the Lotus Scorpion II.

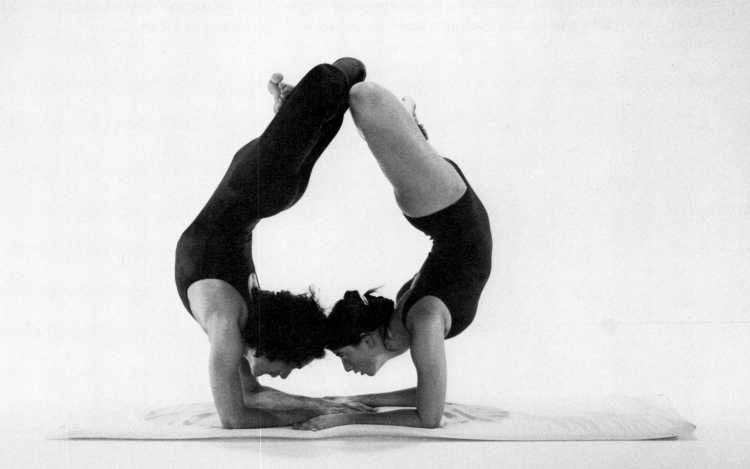

THE LOTUS SCORPION II

When you are proficient at the Lotus Scorpion I, you may progress to this pose. Both partners place their hands in a line on the floor, with one partner's hands inside the other's. Lift both heads up until they are touching, if possible. Then raise the legs and come into the Lotus. Bring the knees together while extending your spine and firmly tucking the tailbone down. Be very careful and attentive in this pose so you don't fall or knock each other over.

BENEFITS: This pose is an intense and invigorating back bend. It tones the whole body and requires great concentration.

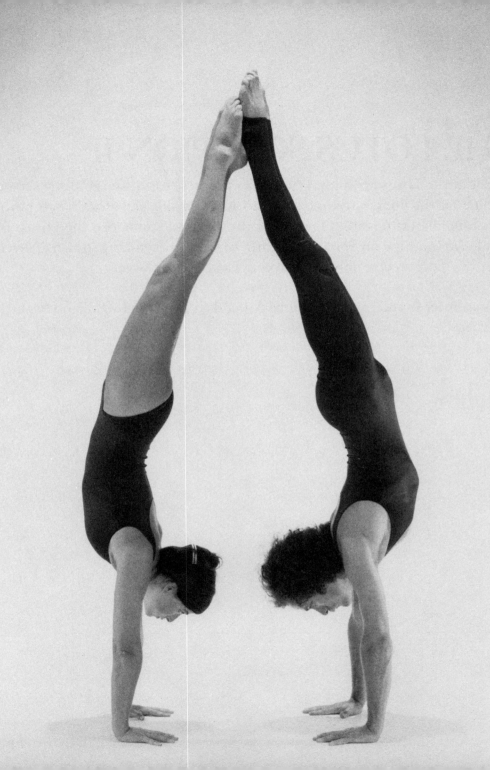

☀ THE HAND STAND

Before attempting the double Hand Stand both partners should be proficient in the pose alone. Practice against a wall to improve strength and balance. First one partner comes into the Hand Stand and gets steady. Then the second partner comes into the pose about two feet away. Slowly arch back until your feet meet and press lightly together. You may carefully and evenly increase the amount of pressure on the feet to make the pose more stable, but be sure to tell your partner before you release and come down!

BENEFITS: The Hand Stand is wonderful for strengthening the upper parts of the body. Regular practice will make the wrists, arms, shoulders, and pectoral muscles strong and improve balance and stamina. The Hand Stand is fun, exhilarating, and energizing.

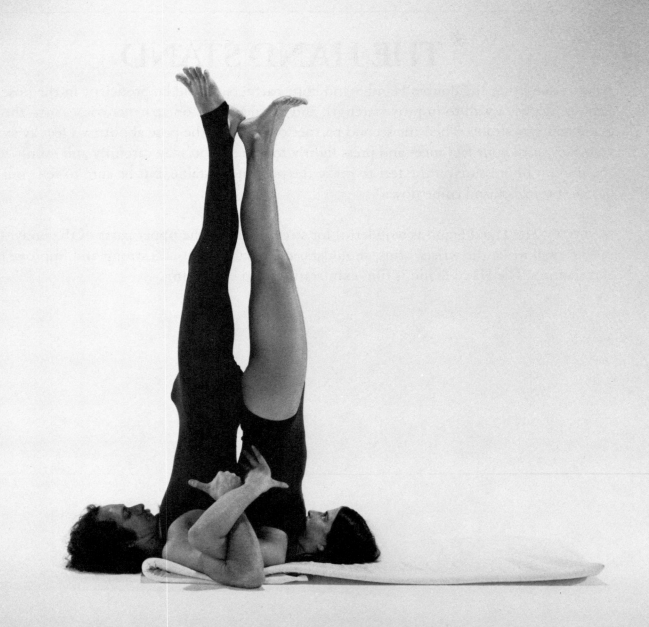

THE SHOULDER STAND

The double Shoulder Stand requires a bit of maneuvering to get into, but the benefits of mutual support are well worth the effort. Do the pose on a mat, blanket, or carpet. First, one partner comes into the Shoulder Stand, raising up onto the neck and shoulders and supporting the trunk and legs vertically with the hands on the back. Then the other comes into the Plow (page 153) a few feet behind, places the hands on the floor by the shoulders, and pushes and slides until your backs are pressed together. The second partner then raises the legs up to meet the first partner's. Interlock arms as shown and support your backs with your hands, keeping torsos vertical as you ascend. Make sure the head and neck are straight—not twisted or tilted to one side. If the neck is being pulled too tightly, put extra padding under the shoulders and arms only (not under the neck). Hold the pose three to five minutes, breathing deeply and evenly. In order to balance out the stretch of the upper back and neck the Shoulder Stand should be followed by the Cross-Bound Lotus (page 203), the Fish (page 163), or the Forward Fold (page 167).

BENEFITS: The Shoulder Stand, the queen of Yoga positions, provides the numerous benefits of inverted poses. Gravity drains stagnant blood out of the legs and the thyroid and parathyroid glands are regulated. The pose is a great tension-reliever because the neck receives increased blood flow and is stretched and relaxed. The Shoulder Stand is recommended for those with varicose veins or tired, cramped, or aching legs. It tones and rejuvenates the whole body, lowers blood pressure, and has a general relaxation effect.

THE SHOULDER STAND, LEG MOVEMENTS

Assume the Shoulder Stand pose and lower one leg to the floor. You may both lower the same leg or opposite legs for different effects. The heels of the upward legs are pressed together for leverage. Hold for a few moments and then change legs.

BENEFITS: These movements strengthen the back and stomach muscles. The up-and-down stretching action relieves tenseness in the legs and increases circulation in them after the Shoulder Stand.

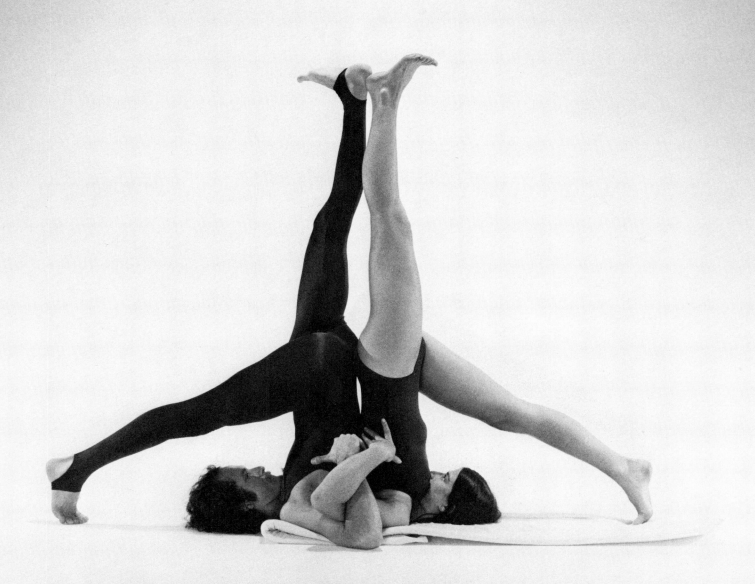

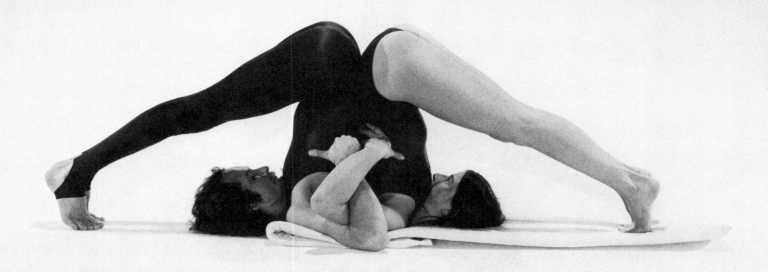

THE PLOW

From the Shoulder Stand, lower one leg at a time over the head to the floor. (When your back and stomach muscles are strong enough, lower both legs in synchronization with your partner.) If your feet will not reach the floor, support them on the seat of a low chair or a small box. Then, pressing your backs against each other, push with the toes to get more lift and to roll the hips closer together. Hold, breathing evenly. If your feet are comfortably resting on the floor, then together walk the legs clockwise and then counterclockwise, holding a few moments at each maximum point.

BENEFITS: Lowering the legs from the Shoulder Stand to the Plow greatly strengthens the abdominal and back muscles. Rolling the hips together allows you to put traction on the lumbar region, thus lengthening the spine. The Plow gives most of the benefits of the Shoulder Stand and is an easy pose for relaxing and recharging the body.

THE BRIDGE

Come into the Plow. One remains in the Plow while the other arches back until the feet rest on the Plow partner's legs. One partner holds the Plow firmly while the other presses down with the feet to get more lift in the spine. Hold and stretch, then change.

BENEFITS: The Bridge movements are used to increase the mobility of the back muscles and vertebrae. By slowly lowering down into position and lifting up again, the back and stomach are strengthened.

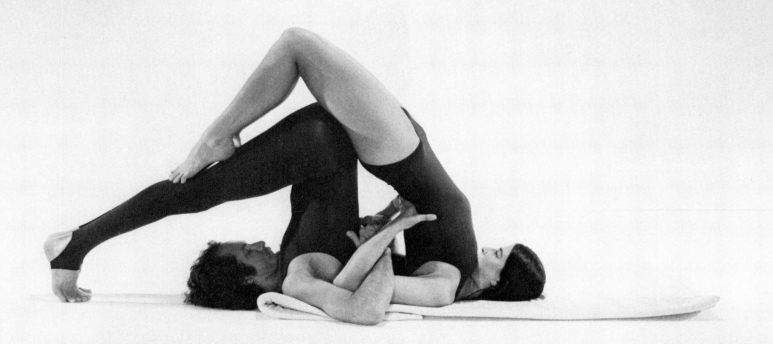

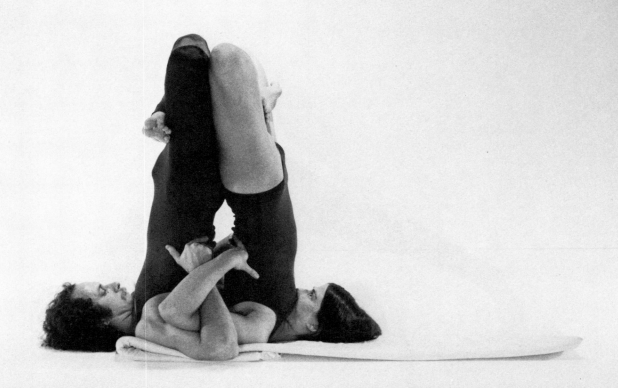

THE LOTUS SHOULDER STAND

From the Shoulder Stand, bring one foot at a time onto the thighs into the Lotus or Half Lotus. If necessary, use your hands to pull the feet into place. Press knees with your partner, tuck your tailbone under, and lift. Hold, breathe deeply and rhythmically, then bend forward into the Folded Lotus on the following page.

BENEFITS: This pose combines the benefits of the Shoulder Stand and the Lotus. It opens the front of the pelvis, assists you in getting a good vertical lift, and is very stable.

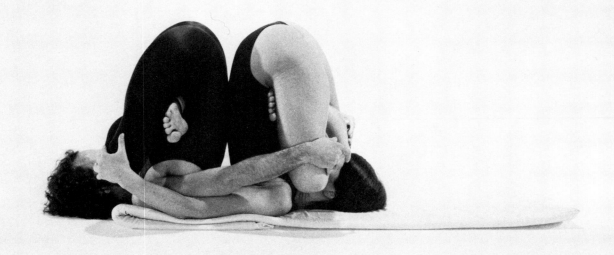

☀ THE FOLDED LOTUS
SHOULDER STAND

From the Lotus Shoulder Stand, bend forward at the hips, bringing the folded knees as close to the chest as possible. Then reach back to clasp each other's knees and pull them in. Press your backs together, lifting your spines straight. You may change from this pose directly to the Fish (page 163) by sliding apart, clasping arms, and pressing your folded legs together.

BENEFITS: This pose gives a concentrated stretch to the buttock muscles and lumbar region.

☀ THE LOTUS BRIDGE

Come into the Shoulder Stand on a mat back to back about four feet apart. The first partner lowers the feet into the Bridge (page 154), tucking the toes under the other partner's shoulder blades. The second partner comes into the Lotus and bends back, gently lowering onto the first partner's legs. Keep your tailbones tucked. Hold a few moments, allowing the spine to stretch. Then raise back to the Shoulder Stand and change positions.

BENEFITS: This pose strengthens and flexes the neck, back, stomach, and wrists. It gives a gentle, supported back bend for the partner in the Lotus position.

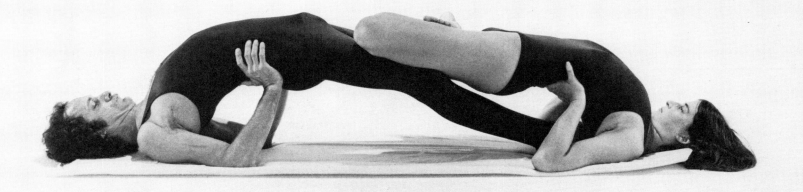

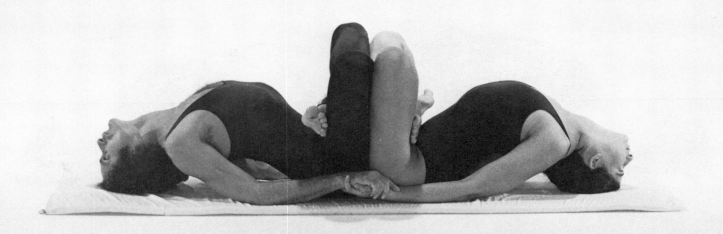

THE FISH

This is a double version of the Fish, a pose used by Yogis to float in the water. On a mat or a carpet, come into the Half Lotus or Lotus and slide the backs of the legs against your partner. Press down with the elbows and arch the chest up, placing the top of the head onto the mat. Clasp hands or wrists and pull to increase the lift in the chest.

BENEFITS: The Fish complements the Shoulder Stand by stretching the neck and upper back in opposite directions. It opens the chest and relieves tightness in the bronchial tubes, thereby increasing breathing capacity. The thyroid and parathyroid glands are toned and roundness in the shoulders is corrected.

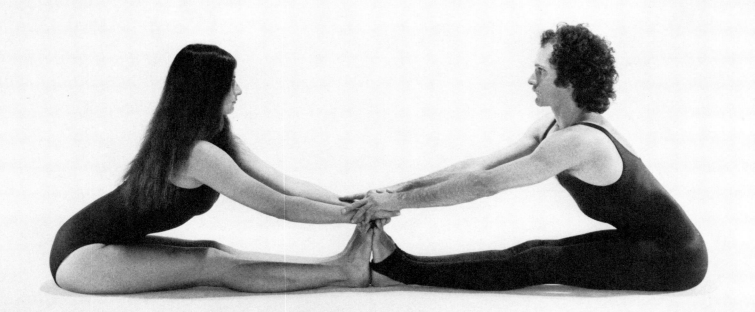

THE HALF FORWARD FOLD

Sit with feet pressed evenly together at a right angle to ankles. Exhale slowly as you extend forward and hold your partner's hands or wrists. Use the pull from your partner to lift your chest and elongate your spine all the way from the tailbone to the head. Pay special attention to stretching the inside of the legs forward and pushing against the inside edge of your partner's sole. Keep your legs straight with knees pressed down. Breathe rhythmically, exhaling into the stretch, and hold the pose for at least three minutes.

BENEFITS: The Half Forward Fold is one of the great Yogic positions and has numerous benefits. The sedentary pattern of modern life causes the muscles of the legs and back to shrink, which puts pressure on the nerves and skeleton. Forward bending, by lengthening all the muscles, ligaments, and tendons from the feet to the head, creates freedom and mobility in the body. The sciatic nerves are stretched, tension is released, cramps (muscular and menstrual) are prevented, and posture is improved. This pose helps to lower high blood pressure, improve digestion and circulation, soothe the nervous system, and quiet the brain.

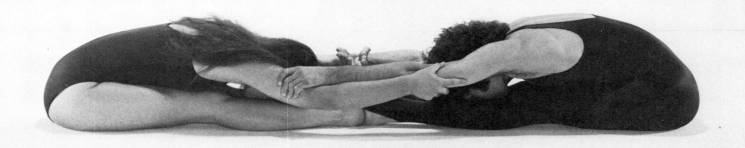

THE FORWARD FOLD

Follow the instructions for the Half Forward Fold, but after holding, continue to fold forward, sliding your hands up your partner's arms. Hold the pose, using the push against the feet and the pull on the arms to increase the extension and straighten the back.

BENEFITS: The pressing of feet and pulling of arms with your partner lifts the chest and puts emphasis on stretching the back and hamstring muscles.

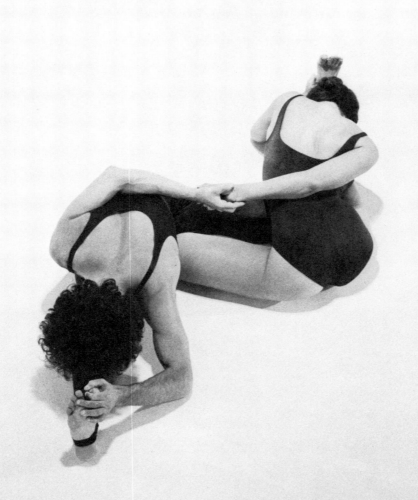

THE HALF-BOUND FORWARD FOLD

Sit next to your partner, facing in opposite directions with your legs extended. Draw your inside leg up into your groin and keep your knee on the floor. Slide close enough to your partner for your shinbones to touch. Bring your outside arm around behind your back to grip hands with your partner. Sit up straight, inhaling. Then, exhaling, bend forward and catch your toes. Hold, come up, and turn around on your hips to face the other direction and do the other side.

BENEFITS: This pose provides all the benefits of forward bending. In addition, the clasping of hands behind the back assists in keeping the torso pressed down and the back from rounding.

THE RECLINING
FORWARD FOLD I

Sit back to back and have your partner come into the Forward Fold. Recline back and reach overhead to grab your partner's toes or arms. Keep your feet flexed and allow your back to stretch, pressing your folded partner down. Hold positions for a few minutes, then sit up and change smoothly so that the forward-folding partner reclines and the reclining partner folds forward.

BENEFITS: The reclining partner receives a gentle, supported back bend that opens the spine, intercostal muscles, shoulders, and armpits. The folded partner is pushed down and forward into the pose, which allows relaxation and muscle stretching.

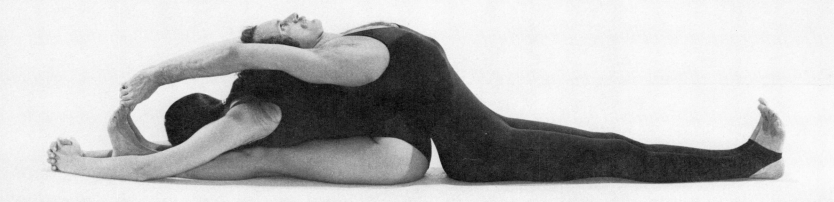

THE RECLINING
FORWARD FOLD II

Follow the instructions for Reclining Forward Fold I, this time with the reclining partner sitting in the Half Lotus or Lotus position. The folded partner reaches back and joins hands gently over the other's stomach, as shown. Hold, and then change so that the reclining partner extends the legs and bends forward as the folded partner crosses the legs and reclines.

BENEFITS: The reclining partner is able to sit in the Half Lotus or Lotus and receive an even stretch along the spine. The folded partner is pressed down into a forward bend and may also gently massage the other partner's stomach to aid digestion and elimination.

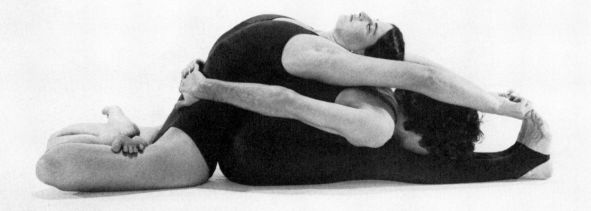

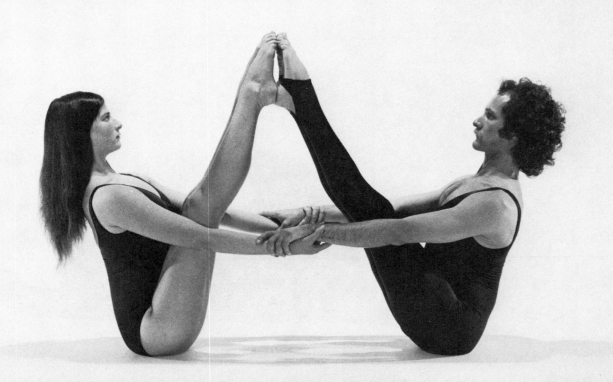

THE ASCENDED
SOLE BALANCE

Sit facing your partner with knees bent and legs drawn in. Hold hands, balance on your buttocks, and press your soles together. Ascend the soles, straightening your legs. Pull against your partner's hands, press your feet together, pointing the toes, and raise your chest.

BENEFITS: This pose improves balance and stretches the legs, ankles, and insteps.

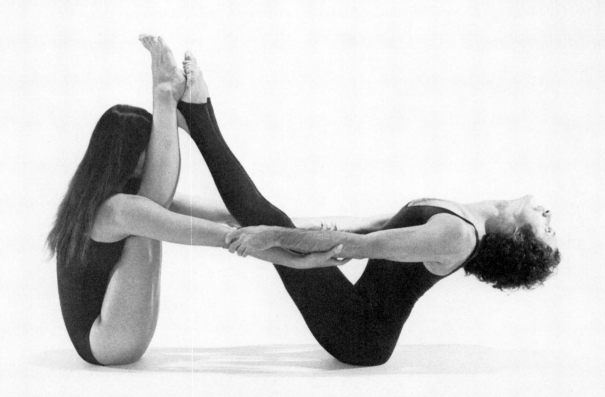

THE VISE

Come into the Ascended Sole pose. One partner slides the feet down to press firmly on the other partner's Achilles tendons or calves. This partner arches back, pulling the other forward to press legs against body and head. Both partners should keep spines extended as much as possible. Hold, then change.

BENEFITS: In this pose one partner is able to get a good backward arch while pulling the other forward. The viselike stretch gives the forward-bending partner an intense pull, more so than when doing the pose alone.

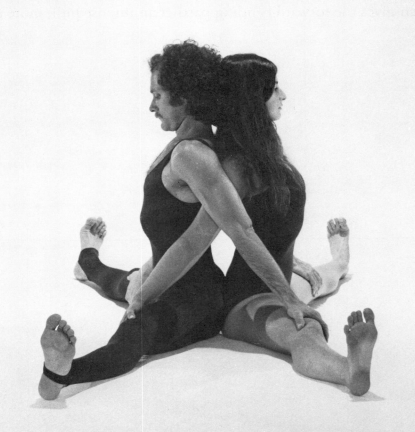

THE STRADDLE SPLIT LIFT

Sit back to back with your legs spread in the straddle split, as shown. Reach back and hold your partner's inner thighs. Pull gently as you lift your chest. Keep the feet at right angles to the floor.

BENEFITS: This pose gives an easy stretch along the legs, inner thighs, and back, preparing you for more advanced positions.

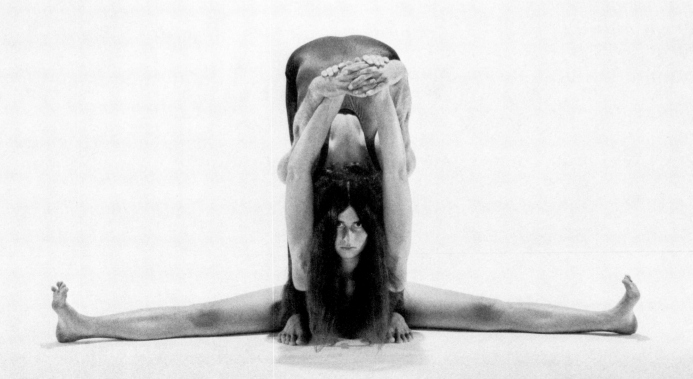

☀ THE DETENT

Sit in the straddle split with your feet at right angles to the floor and bend forward. Your partner stands over you, feet at your groin with heels pressing your thighs open. (The pose can be made easier by standing with the feet behind the thighs.) Then your partner folds forward with hands clasped high overhead and you arch up to hold hands as shown. Breathe evenly.

BENEFITS: *Detent* means to stretch one mechanical part tightly in relation to another. The inner leg and thigh muscles of the split partner are lengthened, full mobility is brought to the shoulders, the torso is elongated, and the chest is opened.

☀ THE SPLITS

Come into the Splits facing each other, supporting the weight of the body with the arms as you ease onto the floor, and press your left feet evenly together as you slide the right legs back. Fold forward as far as possible. Then clasp each other's arms and pull into the stretch. Hold, then change to the other side.

BENEFITS: The Splits give a powerful stretch along the legs, thighs, groin, and hips. The tendons, ligaments, and muscles are elongated, tension is released, and circulation is improved, preventing leg cramps and increasing mobility.

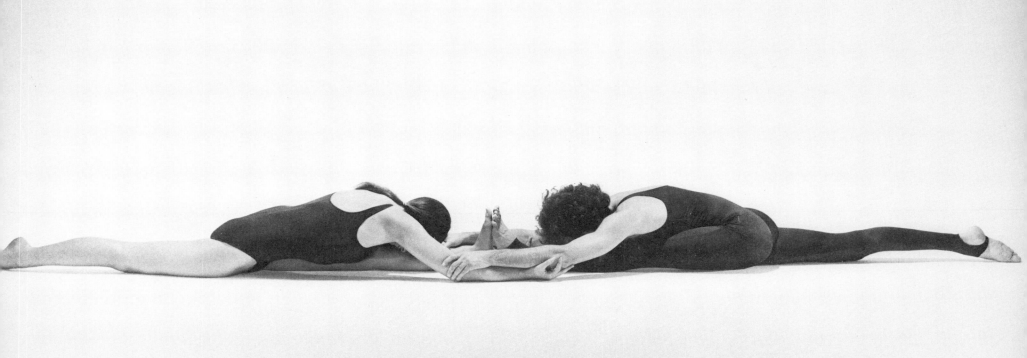

☀ THE STRADDLE BOND

Sit in the straddle split facing one another about six feet apart. Hold hands and, exhaling, extend forward, sliding your hands up your partner's arms as far as you can. Maintain a gentle pull on each other.

BENEFITS: This pose stretches the muscles of the groin, inner legs, and thighs. These muscles tend to shorten from lack of use and this posture restores freedom and mobility to the pelvis and legs.

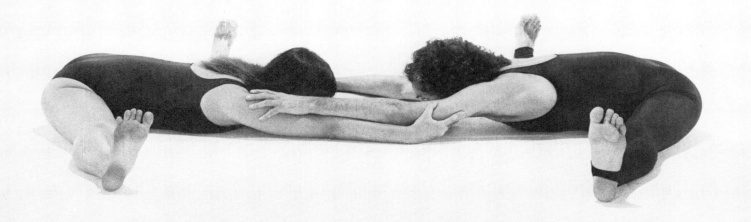

☀ THE STAR TORTOISE

Sit back to back in the straddle split. Bend your torsos forward, bend your knees slightly, and slide your hands under your knees to hook fingers with your partner. Straighten your legs, extend your spine, and flex your feet back.

BENEFITS: This pose produces all the effects of forward bending and straddle split, with the added benefits obtained from being locked into position by placing your arms under your legs.

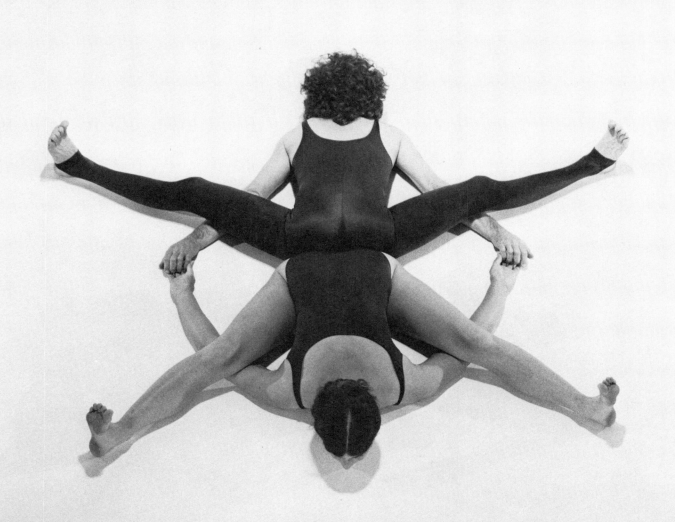

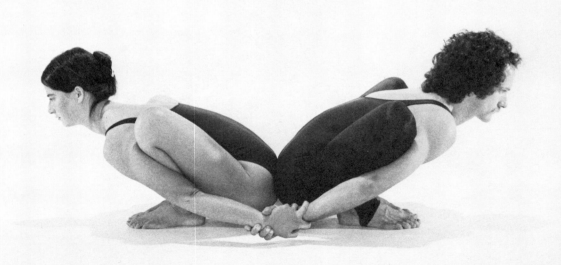

THE FROG LINK

Squat back to back with your feet together and press against your partner's buttocks. Spread your knees and sink your torso between your thighs. Reach back and around to clasp your partner's wrists. Then press your triceps against your shinbones and use your partner's pull to extend forward from the tailbone to the head. Keep your heels down if possible.

BENEFITS: The Frog Link stretches the Achilles tendons and inner legs. Its major effect is to relieve compression in the lower back and sacrum area, which aids elimination.

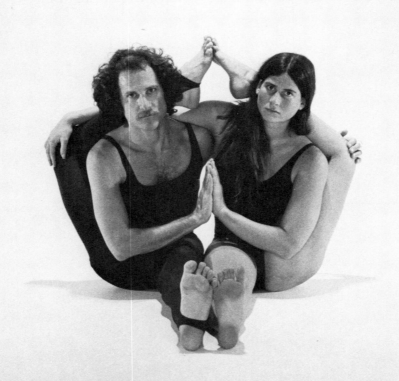

☀ THE PENTAGON

Sit alongside each other and pull your outside leg over your shoulder, placing it behind your head and neck. Bend your head back to lock the leg in place. Then bring the outside hands and feet together in *namaste* (joined palm salute) and the inside arms around behind to hold your partner's knee. Sit up and lean back, stretching the bent leg. Keep your breathing even. After holding the pose, clasp the foot of your extended leg and fold forward, exhaling. Allow the back leg to push you down into the stretch. Hold, then change sides.

BENEFITS: This pose gives an intense stretch to the hamstrings and creates mobility in the hip joints. The lumbar area is stretched, and as you fold forward, the push of the back leg helps to lengthen the leg muscles.

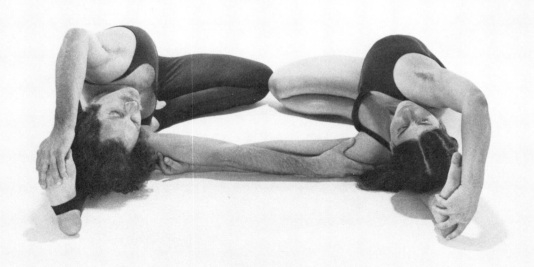

THE ROLLED FOLD

Sit alongside your partner, about three feet apart, with legs outstretched. Bring your inside foot to your groin, sliding the leg back to create a wide angle between your thighs. Your partner does the same and then you touch knees, keeping your extended legs parallel. Exhaling, revolve your torso toward your partner, fold forward, and grab your front foot, pulling with your arm to keep the lower side of your trunk extended. Then hold inside arms, pulling on each other to increase the twist and keep your chests rolled upward. Hold, then change sides.

BENEFITS: Pulling your partner gives an excellent twist that relieves lower-back pain. It also stretches all the leg muscles and opens the shoulders and intercostal muscles, which increases your ability to breathe deeply to fill the lungs.

THE CROSS GATE

Kneel about six feet apart side by side, extend one leg, and press the outside edges of your feet together. Clasp the lower hands and bend in toward each other. Stretch the upper arms together to hold hands and keep the torso rotated up. Turn the head to look up while keeping the hips and chest facing forward, as shown. The correct movement is obtained by lifting and pulling outward with the torso, which stretches the arms taut. Hold and then change sides.

BENEFITS: This pose gives an intense lateral stretch. It removes stiffness from the back and shoulders.

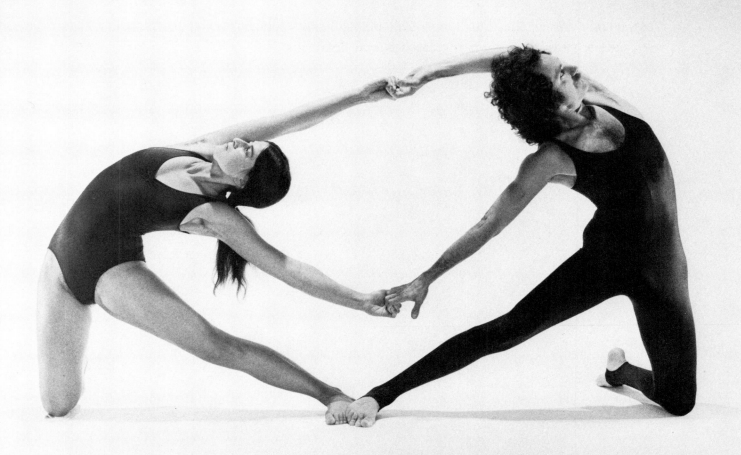

THE SHOOTING STAR I

Sit side by side with inside legs touching. Place the outside foot to the groin or on the thigh in the Half Lotus. Twist toward each other, reaching with the outside arm to clasp each other's foot. Extend the inside arms up, palms pressed, and lift, pulling each other into the twist. Look up at the hands. Hold the pose, breathing into the stretch, then change sides.

BENEFITS: This aesthetic and enjoyable pose gives a stretching twist to the spinal column, which removes tension and brings increased lateral flexibility.

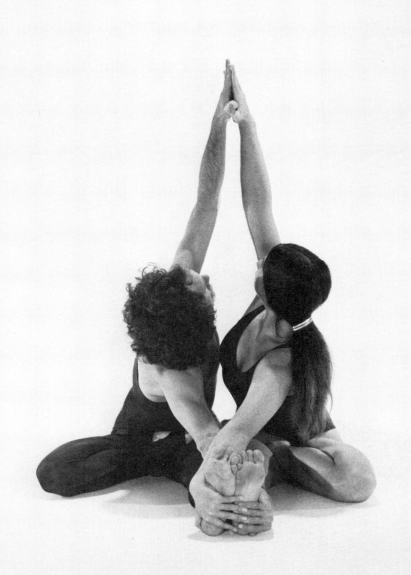

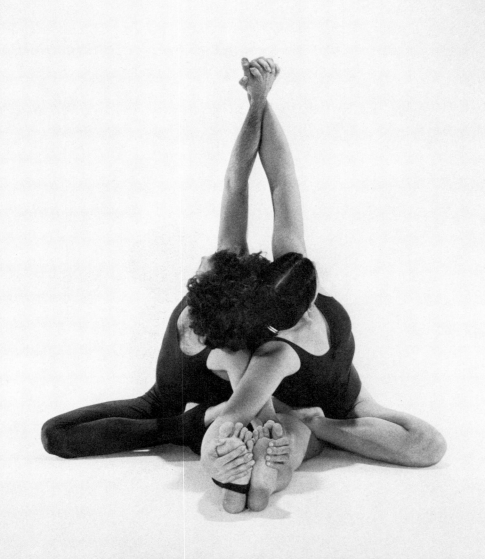

THE SHOOTING STAR II

Sit side by side with inside legs touching. Place the outside foot at the groin or on the thigh in the Half Lotus. Twist away from each other, reaching with the inside arm to clasp each other's foot. Extend the outside arms up to hold crossed hands and press your backs together and look up. Pull and lift each other into the twist. Hold the pose, breathing into the stretch, then change sides.

BENEFITS: This pose removes tension in the inner legs and works the same muscle sets as the Rolled Fold, but in a different way.

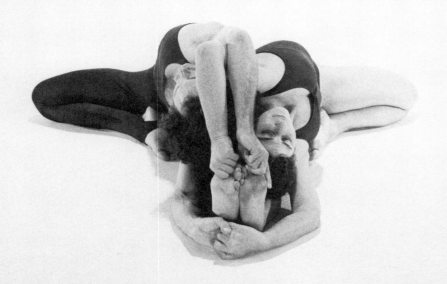

THE STARSHIP

Sit alongside your partner with legs touching. Bend the outside foot to the groin, sliding the leg back to create a wide angle between the thighs. Rotate the torso to face away from your partner and bend sideways over the extended leg. Use the lower arm to reach under the feet and hook fingers with your partner, pulling to extend the lower trunk. (Loop a belt or rope over the feet if you cannot reach them.) Then bring the other arm over to clasp your partner's foot and look up. Push against each other and pull with the arms to stretch and twist into position. Hold, breathing rhythmically, then change.

BENEFITS: The interlocking of arms and pressing of shoulders with your partner allows you to get a full extension and twist. This position gives a rotating lateral stretch to the spine. It also improves digestion and elimination.

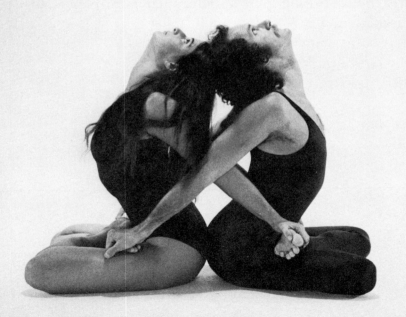

THE CROSS-BOUND LOTUS

Sit back to back in the Lotus position. Reach back with both arms and grab your partner's feet. Lift the chest, arch the back, touch heads, and look up. (Use the Half Lotus or Cross-Legged position if you are unable to do the Lotus.)

BENEFITS: By using your partner to pull and lift, you get a good extension in the upper spine. The chest and intercostal muscles are opened and tension in the thoracic and cervical region is released. This is a good pose to follow the Shoulder Stand (page 149) because it relieves neck tension.

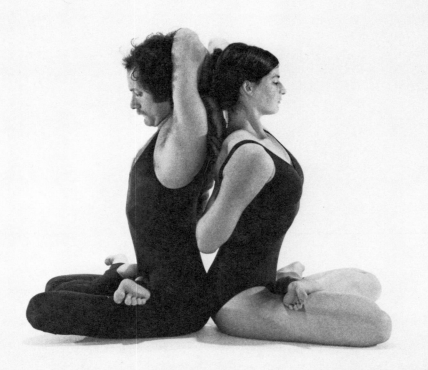

THE WARRIOR

This pose resembles a warrior reaching back to pull arrows out of his quiver. Sit back to back in the Lotus or Cross-Legged position. Both partners raise their left arms, bend them behind the head, and clasp each other's right hand, which is bent low behind the back, as shown. Then you pull each other's upper arm down. Hold, then change arms.

BENEFITS: This pose stretches the triceps, pulls the armpits open, and brings full mobility to the shoulders. It helps to prevent bursitis.

THE LINKED LOTUS BALANCE

Sit in the Lotus or Half Lotus facing your partner. Slide your hands through your legs and in front of your feet. If you are unable to do this, bring your arms around your thighs instead. Clasp hands or wrists with your partner as you sit up straight. Then rock back and balance.

BENEFITS: This pose flexes the knees and ankles and improves balance.

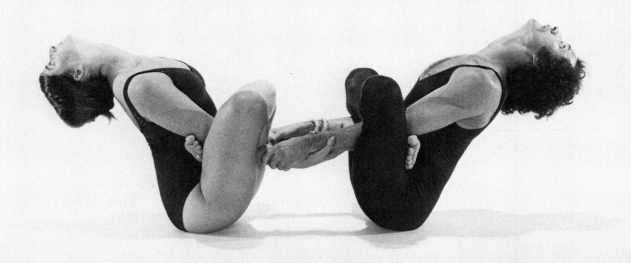

☀ THE HUGGING LOTUS

Sit facing each other in the Lotus or Half Lotus. Brace with arms on the floor behind you and fold the Lotus up, bringing the knees to the chest. Slide together, balance, and reach around to hold each other's back. Pull on each other, pressing the Lotuses in and lifting the chest.

BENEFITS: Pressing together in this pose gives a good stretch that expands the lumbar area and backs of the thighs. To stay balanced you must work your back muscles, which will strengthen and tone them.

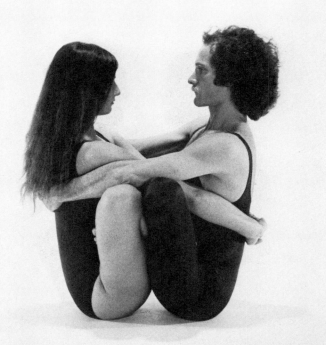

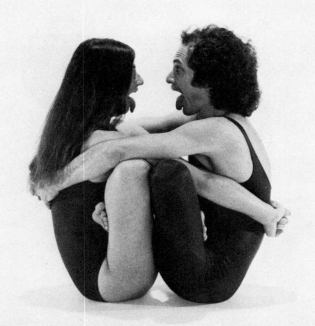

☀ THE ROARING LOTUS

Sit in the Hugging Lotus pose. Inhale, and simultaneously open the mouth, stretch the tongue down, roll the eyes up, tense the whole body, and quickly, forcibly exhale through the mouth. Hold the tensed position with the breath out for fifteen seconds. Then inhale, take a few breaths, and repeat. If you practice until you can do this procedure instantaneously, the effects will be increased.

BENEFITS: In this pose you will feel a surge of energy. The Roaring Lotus massages and brings blood to the throat, keeping it in good health. And it lightens the spirit!

THE LOTUS MOUNTAIN

Sit back to back in the Lotus or Half Lotus on a mat. Raise up on your knees, walk them in close to your partner, and press the buttocks together. Extend the arms overhead, hold hands, and lift.

BENEFITS: This pose improves balance, strengthens the knees, and opens the shoulder joints.

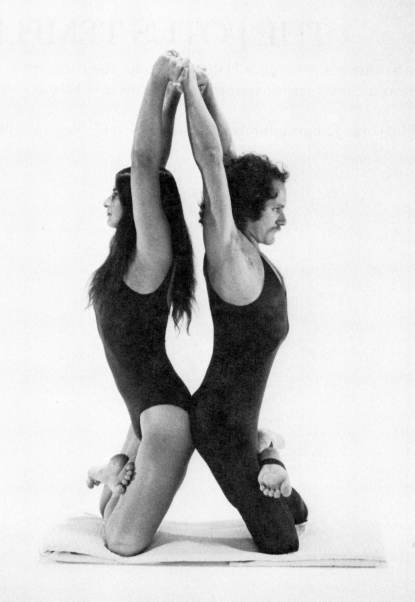

THE LOTUS TEMPLE

Sit facing each other in the Lotus or Half Lotus about three feet apart. Push up onto your knees, extend the arms up, press against your partner's palms, and balance.

BENEFITS: The Lotus Temple improves balance and strengthens the knees.

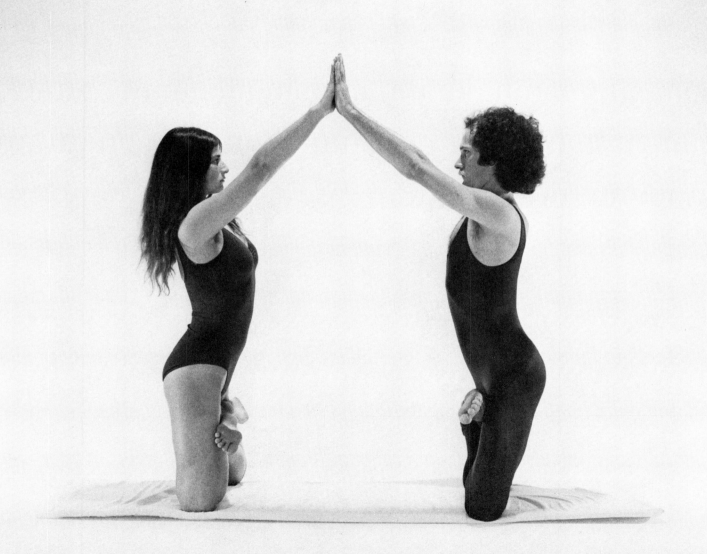

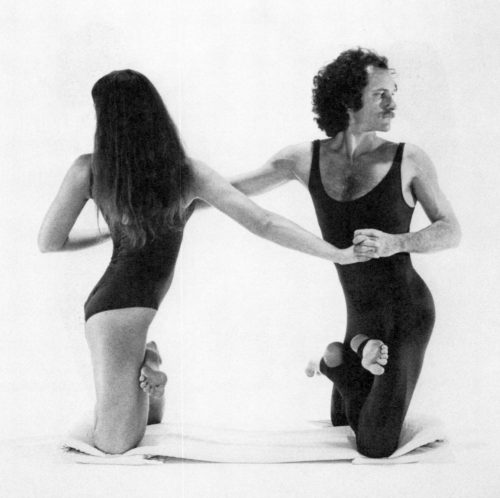

THE DANCING LOTUS

Sit in the Lotus or Half Lotus about three feet apart. Raise up on your knees and hold hands at waist level. Push and pull each other into a twist. Hold and stretch, then change directions several times.

BENEFITS: The rotating movement warms up the back muscles and relieves compression. It brings lateral flexibility to the spine.

THE LOTUS LION

Sit in the Lotus or Half Lotus about six feet apart. Stand up on your knees, place your hands on the floor with fingertips pointing back, and support your trunk with straight arms. Let your hips sink down as far as possible. Then, inhale and at the same moment do all of the following: open your mouth, extend your tongue out and down, roll your eyes up, and exhale through your mouth with great force.

BENEFITS: Supporting the weight of the torso and letting the hips drop relieves pain in the lower spine and tailbone. This pose opens the pelvis. It produces a surge of energy and strengthens the throat and tongue, increasing blood circulation in these areas. The forearms and wrists are stretched and toned.

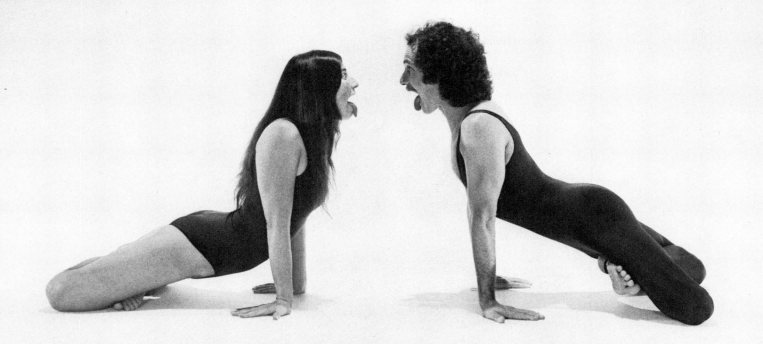

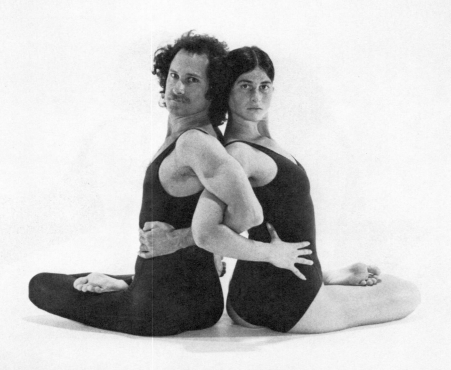

THE ELBOW TWIST

Sit side by side in the Lotus or Cross-Legged position, facing in the same direction. With the hips and sides of the thighs touching, extend your inside arms and hold your partner's inside knee. Twist toward the outside and hook elbows, pressing the shoulders together, and exhale into the stretch. Repeat on the other side.

BENEFITS: This pose is easy and beneficial for both beginning and advanced students. The hips are kept flat on the floor, which aligns the spine properly. The pressed shoulders and elbow lock provide support and assist you in getting a good twist and extension.

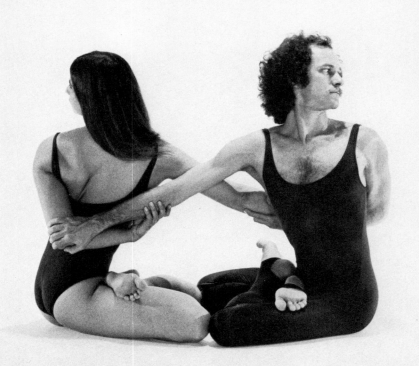

THE LOTUS TWIST

Sit facing your partner in the Lotus or Half Lotus with your knees touching. Twist to the left and bend your left arm behind your back. Reach out with your right hand to clasp your partner's left arm or elbow. Lift your chest and keep your spine vertical as you pull each other around into the twist. Hold, then change sides.

BENEFITS: The Lotus Twist is easy for most people to do, yet it gives a very good twist to the spine. The placement of the arm behind the back assists in keeping the chest lifted, the spine straight, and the shoulders back and open. By pulling against each other, the partners can twist more and get increased benefit.

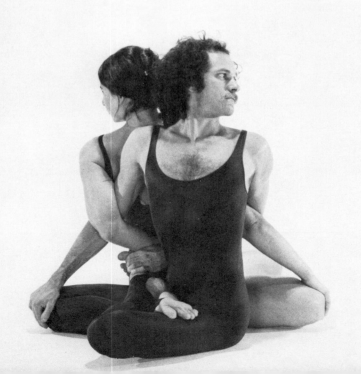

THE INTERTWINED TWIST

Sit side by side in a Lotus or Cross-Legged position, facing in opposite directions so that your right hips touch. As you twist toward the left, extend your right arm and hold your right knee. Bend your left arm around behind your back, over your partner's extended right arm, and clasp your left foot or inside thigh. Hold firmly, keep the spine erect, and pull each other around as you straighten your extended arm. Exhale into the twist and hold, breathing evenly. Then change sides.

BENEFITS: The Intertwined Twist provides all the regular benefits of the twist poses. In addition, the arm lock increases your ability to rotate laterally. Each intertwined partner gets a twist with the spine in correct alignment. The shoulders are kept back and open.

❋ THE PUSH-ME, PULL-YOU TWIST I

Sit erect facing your partner and draw your right foot up. Place it outside your extended leg, keeping your right knee vertical. Slide closer together until your raised knees are touching. Twist toward the right and extend your left arm over your knee while propping up your torso from behind with your right hand on the floor. Then fold your right arm behind your back and hold your partner's left arm, as shown. Turn your head to the right, sit up straight, and pull on each other, exhaling into the twist. Hold, then change sides.

BENEFITS: This pose is fantastic for adjusting the spine and releasing tension. The push/pull action of the partners assists in getting a full twist and moving areas that are difficult to reach alone. Twisting relieves pressure on the nerves, increases nerve efficiency, and alleviates back pain. The pose rebalances the spine after intense back bends or forward bends.

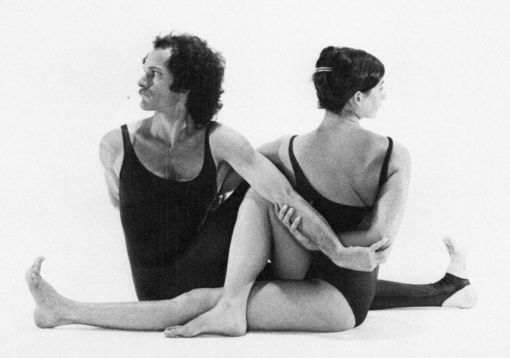

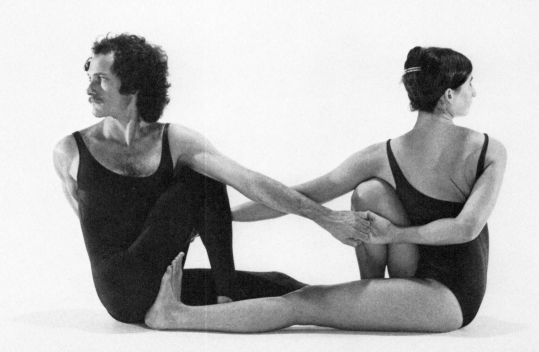

THE PUSH-ME, PULL-YOU TWIST II

Sit up straight facing your partner and draw your right foot into your groin, keeping your knee vertical. Twist toward the right and put your left arm over your knee, while propping up your torso from behind with your right hand on the floor. Then grab your partner's right hand with your left, as shown. The foot of the extended leg is kept against your partner's thigh as you push and pull each other, exhaling into the twist. Repeat on the other side.

BENEFITS: This pose gives a more intense rotation than the Push-Me, Pull-You Twist I.

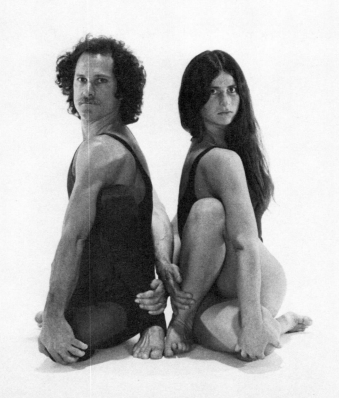

✺ THE SPINAL TWIST

Sit side by side and bend the inside leg into a Half Lotus and sit on the foot. Then bring your outside foot over the bent leg and pull your heel close to your hip, keeping your knee as vertical as possible. Now twist toward your raised knee, reaching around behind your back to grab your partner's ankle. Lift your torso up straight, extend your inside arm over the raised knee, and hold your lower knee. Exhale into the twist, turning your head in the opposite direction the spine is twisting. Hold, then change sides.

BENEFITS: The Spinal Twist is a great Yogic pose. It aligns the vertebrae, relieves compression, and develops lateral flexibility. It also improves digestion and elimination. Turning the head against the twist of the spine extends the neck and releases pressure on the cervical vertebrae.

NAMASTE!

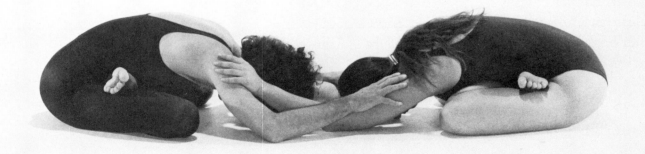

Suggested Practice Sessions

The book is arranged in groupings of poses—standing poses, assisting poses, back bends, inverted poses, forward bends, sitting poses, and twists. There are many possible sequences to follow in practice, and a few are suggested below. Advanced students may start at the beginning of the book and follow the poses as they are presented.

Standing poses strengthen and tone the whole body and over a period of time prepare you for more difficult movements. The standing poses in Double Yoga provide a full range of movements and stretches and can give you a complete workout. Standing poses can be practiced at the beginning or end of a session.

Assisting poses give you the opportunity to aid your partner in achieving a particular stretch or movement or to strengthen a weak area of the body. Assisting poses can be used whenever necessary.

Back bends stimulate the nervous system, counteract the effects of gravity, increase the flow of energy, and bring clarity to the mind. They require concentration and careful practice and should be done when you are fresh—at the beginning of the session after thoroughly warming up. Back bends should be followed by forward bends and twists to remove any residual tension and balance and return the spine to normal.

Forward bends relax and stretch the muscles and soothe the nervous system. They relieve any cramps or tightness accumulated throughout the day or in other poses, and improve posture and body alignment. Forward bends may be practiced at any time during a session.

Twists release pressure on the spinal nerves and align the vertebrae. They are used to balance the spine after back bends and after intense forward bending. The twisting poses can be done during a session as they appear in the book and at the end of a session to release any residual tension.

Sitting poses include back bends, forward bends, twists, and balancing positions. They may be included in the appropriate groupings or practiced in sequence together.

Note: Times are for each side in poses with two directions.

Beginning Session I

POSE	TIME
Tree I	30 sec.–1 min.
Triangle	30 sec.
Fence	30 sec.
Hero II	30 sec.
Suspension Bridge	1 min.
Pump	1 min.
Chair	30 sec. (2 times)
Hip-Supported Back Stretch	30 sec.
Reclining Forward Fold I	1 min. (2 times)
Half Forward Fold	2 min.
Ascended Sole Balance	30 sec. (2 times)
Straddle Split Lift	1 min.
Shoulder Stand	3–5 min.
Cross-Bound Lotus or Fish (do in Cross-Legged position)	30 sec.
Forward Fold	3–5 min.
Elbow Twist	30 sec. (2 times)
Namaste	
Relaxation	5–15 min.

Beginning Session II

POSE	TIME
Suspension Bridge	1–2 min.
Triangle	30 sec.

POSE	TIME
Extended Hero	30 sec.
Linked Forward Fold	1 min.
Tree II	1 min.
Chair	30 sec.
Shoulder Stand	3 min.
Shoulder Stand, Leg Movements	2 min.
Cross-Bound Lotus or Fish (do in Cross-Legged position)	30 sec.
Back Stretcher I	1 min.
Half Forward Fold	3 min.
Lotus Twist	1 min.
Namaste	
Relaxation	5–10 min.

Intermediate Session I

POSE	TIME
Triangle	1 min.
Big Toe	30 sec.
Royal Crown	30 sec.
Twisting Fence	30 sec.
Hero I	45 sec.
Pyramid	30 sec.
Full Moon	30 sec.
Extended Hero	45 sec.
Twisting Triangle	30 sec.
Linked Forward Fold	1–2 min.
Split Mushroom	1 min.
Ankle Lock I or II	1 min.
Chair	30 sec.

POSE	TIME	POSE	TIME
Arm-Supported Back Bend to Arm-Supported Forward Fold	back and forth 3 times holding 30 sec. in each	Plow	2 min.
		Bridge	3 times
		Cross-Bound Lotus or Fish	30 sec.
		Lotus Mountain	30 sec.
Belt-Assisted Back Bend	30 sec. (2 times)	Lotus Temple	30 sec.
Fountain	30 sec. (2 times)	Ascended Sole Balance	1–2 min.
Camel	30 sec. (2 times)	Vise	1–2 min.
Crescent Moon I or II	30 sec. (2 times)	Half-Bound Forward Fold	2 min.
Suspension Bridge	1–2 min.	Forward Fold	5 min.
Forward Fold	3–5 min.	Straddle Bond	2 min.
Vise	30 sec.	Shooting Star I and II	30 sec.
Rolled Fold	1 min.	Hero I	1 min.
Shoulder Stand, Leg Movements	5 min.	Pyramid	1 min.
Plow	1 min.	Extended Hero	1 min.
Cross-Bound Lotus or Fish	30 sec.	Full Moon	1 min.
Intertwined Twist	30 sec.	Twisting Triangle	1 min.
Spinal Twist	30 sec.	Suspension Bridge	1 min.
Namaste		Namaste	
Relaxation	5–15 min.	Relaxation	5–15 min.

Intermediate Session II

POSE	TIME
Suspension Bridge	1–2 min.
Linked Forward Fold	2 min.
Rope Extension Stretch	1 min. (2 times)
Cross Gate	30 sec.
Head Stand	3–5 min.
Shoulder Stand	5–10 min.

Advanced Session

POSE	TIME
Triangle	1 min.
Extended Hero	45 sec.
Pyramid	1 min.
Full Moon	45 sec.
Hero Balance	30 sec.
Diamond Hero	30 sec.

POSE	TIME
Twisting Triangle	45 sec.
Twisting Diamond Hero	30 sec.
Twisting Hero	45 sec.
Linked Forward Fold	1–2 min.
Mushroom I	1 min.
Scissors	30 sec.
Standing Tortoise	30 sec.
Hand Stand	30 sec. (2 times)
Archway	30 sec. (3 times)
Camel	30 sec. (3 times)
Arrowhead Scorpion	30 sec.–1 min.
Crescent Moon II	30 sec. (2 times)
Suspension Bridge	1–2 min.
Ankle Lock I	1 min.
Head Stand	5–10 min.
Shoulder Stand	5–10 min.
Lotus Shoulder Stand	2 min.
Folded Lotus Shoulder Stand	1 min.
Plow	3 min.
Fish	45 sec.
Forward Fold	3–5 min.
Rolled Fold	1 min.
Starship	1 min.
Splits	1 min. (2 times)
Push-Me, Pull-You Twist I	45 sec.
Spinal Twist	45 sec.
Namaste	
Relaxation	5–15 min.

Back Bend Emphasis Session

POSE	TIME
Suspension Bridge	2 min.
Ankle Lock I	2 min.
Linked Forward Fold	1 min.
Hand Stand	30 sec. (2 times)
Hip-Supported Back Stretch I	1 min. (2–3 times)
Hip-Supported Back Stretch II	1 min.
Arm-Supported Back Bend to Arm-Supported Forward Fold	back and forth 5–10 times holding each 20 sec.
Diamond Hero	30 sec.
Fountain	30 sec. (3 times)
Archway	30 sec. (3 times)
Belt-Linked Back Bend	30 sec. (5 times)
Camel	30 sec. (4 times)
Crescent Moon I and II	30 sec. (2 times)
Arrowhead Scorpion	30 sec.–1 min.
Lotus Scorpion I	30 sec.–1 min.
Reclining Forward Fold I	1–2 min.
Reclining Forward Fold II	1–2 min.
Frog Link	2 min.
Forward Fold	5 min.
Lotus Twist	1 min.
Shooting Star I	1 min.
Shooting Star II	1 min.
Push-Me, Pull-You Twist I or II	1 min.

POSE	TIME
Head Stand	3–5 min.
Shoulder Stand	5 min.
Folded Lotus Shoulder Stand	2 min.
Plow	2 min.
Bridge	3 times
Fish	45 sec.
Forward Fold	2 min.
Namaste	
Relaxation	5–15 min.

Forward Bend Emphasis Session

POSE	TIME
Suspension Bridge	1–2 min.
Pyramid	1 min.
Linked Forward Fold	1–2 min.
Pump	1–2 min.
Split Mushroom	30 sec.
Mushroom I	30 sec.
Mushroom II	45 sec.
Facing Forward Fold	1 min.
Standing Tortoise	30 sec.
Scissors	30 sec.
Shiva-Shakti	30 sec.

POSE	TIME
Rope Extension Stretch	1 min.
Back Stretcher I and II	2 min.
Forward Pull	1 min.
Half-Bound Forward Fold	1 min.
Vise	1 min.
Forward Fold	5 min.
Splits	1 min. (2 times)
Detent	45 sec.
Straddle Bond	1–2 min.
Star Tortoise	1 min.
Starship	1 min.
Lotus Temple	30 sec.
Dancing Lotus	30 sec.
Lotus Mountain	30 sec.
Warrior	30 sec.
Intertwined Twist	45 sec.
Spinal Twist	1 min.
Head Stand	3–5 min.
Head Stand Folded Lotus, variation	2–4 times
Shoulder Stand	5 min.
Plow	2 min.
Forward Fold	1 min.
Namaste	
Relaxation	5–15 min.

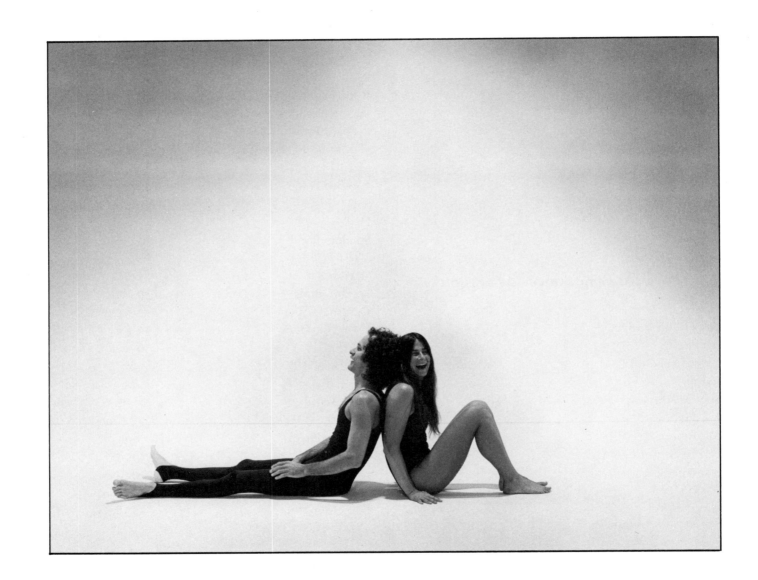

Index of Poses